by M J Clarkson and W B Faull
Department of Veterinary Clinical Science
University of Liverpool

with contributions from

D A R Davies
Department of Animal Husbandry
University of Liverpool
G C Skerritt
Department of Veterinary Preclinical Sciences
University of Liverpool
G S Walton and W R Ward
Department of Veterinary Clinical Science
University of Liverpool

First published as
Notes for the Sheep Clinician
in 1983 by
Liverpool University Press
PO Box 147
Liverpool
L69 3BX

Second edition published 1985
Third edition published 1987

Fourth edition as *A Handbook for the Sheep Clinician*
published 1990

British Library Cataloguing in Publication Data
Clarkson M J
A Handbook for the Sheep Clinician, 4th ed.
1 Sheep – Diseases
I Title II Faull, W B
636.3089 SF968

ISBN 0-85323-346-2

Text processed in
Liverpool University Press
and at
Front End Design Consultants
Liverpool 051-708 7101
Printed by
Redwood Press Limited
Melksham
Wiltshire

" 'The third time he asked, 'Do you love me? – then feed my sheep' "

John 21:17

This book grew out of brief duplicated notes which were given to Final Year veterinary students at the Liverpool Veterinary School.

It was originally designed for undergraduate teaching purposes, where it complements a lecture course and a practical course with individual sick sheep and farm projects. The fourth edition has involved a major revision with not only the updating of information but some increase in depth, bearing in mind the increased involvement of veterinary surgeons with sheep and the introduction of specialist qualifications in Sheep Health and Production by the Royal College of Veterinary Surgeons. We have also included suggestions for further reading, generally from publications readily available in Britain. We have continued to emphasise the practical, clinical aspects of the subject and details of pathology, microbiology, parasitology and many other important areas must be sought elsewhere.

Finally, we have decided that 'handbook' describes this edition better than 'notes'!

Acknowledgements

We are very grateful to all those who originally encouraged us to have our notes published, particularly to Andrew Madel and Andy Eales who had a look at them and made suitable comments! We are also very grateful to Joe Read for advice over the economics section.We are also grateful to many farmers who allowed us to practise on them and their sheep and to the increasing number of veterinary surgeons, especially Agnes Winter and Terry Boundy, who have shared their knowledge with us. This book would never have been completed without the care and efficiency of our secretary, Jean White. We would like to thank Hilary Davies for compiling the index. We are also grateful to John Cox, who represents department authors to the Liverpool University Press, and vice versa, and to the staff of LUP, particularly Robin Bloxsidge, for their expertise and patience!

We have often given some indication of the price of drugs and vaccines, based on information in the October 1989 Index of Veterinary Specialities. In the case of PML products, the price is as stated in IVS; with POM products we have added the usual percentage.

CONTENTS

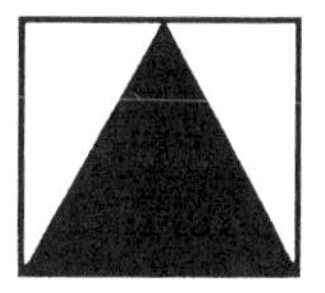

CONTENTS CONTINUED OVERLEAF

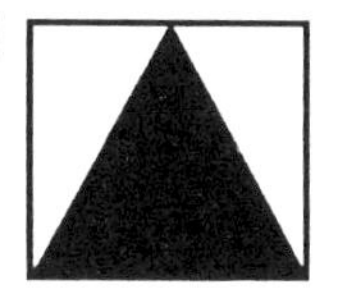

ECONOMICS OF SHEEP PRODUCTION

In order to appreciate the value of individual animals and complete flocks, it is necessary to have some idea as to the main income and costs of the sheep farmer. An appreciation of the economic framework of the industry is an essential background to any veterinary involvement on the sheep farm. The farmer will tend to be more aware of obvious savings such as the value of an individual ewe which might be saved by clinical treatment but preventive health programmes are more financially rewarding to the farmer (and vet) since they influence the overall productivity of the flock.

The Meat and Livestock Commission has over 500 flocks with all systems of management on its recording scheme and publishes data on the production figures and on the finances of these flocks. They also divide the data into 'average', dealing with all the flocks of one system, and 'top-third', based on gross margin per hectare, which shows what improvements are possible and may act as a target for other farmers. It must be recognised that the data for the 'average' flocks are probably much higher than the average of all flocks since the onerous task of keeping accurate records is bound to select for better flocks. These sheets and the *Sheep Yearbook* can be obtained from MLC, Sheep Improvement Services, PO Box 44, Queensway House, Bletchley, MK2 2EF.

An analysis by the MLC of its records from commercial lowland flocks producing lambs for slaughter shows that stocking rate, number of lambs reared, flock replacement costs (ewe longevity), lamb sale price and feed and forage costs are the main performance factors which influence the profitability of the flock.

These factors account for 93% of the superiority of the 'top-third' of their flocks, suggesting that these areas are where the greatest advice is needed. Veterinary advice can improve all these factors e.g. parasite control is crucial to increasing stocking rate and will also influence the time taken to attain marketable weight, which influences the value of the lamb sold. The value of the lamb sold can be influenced most rapidly by changing the terminal ram sire and MLC has carried out large-scale controlled trials with different rams on different commercial ewes.

The ram influences carcase weight and the rate at which lambs mature to the desired fat level and references should be made to MLC results and/or ADAS advisers before recommending a change in ram breed.

A Layman's Guide to the Common Agricultural Policy for Sheep Meat

This section gives an introduction to EEC price structure and reproduces examples of physical and financial production of different types of flock.

This policy, which commenced in 1980 in UK, has increased the income of sheep farmers considerably and has stimulated a steady increase in the national ewe breeding flock from just over 16 million in December 1984 to 20 million in December 1988. An outline of the pricing structure for prime slaughter lambs is given here.

When the EEC Sheepmeat Regime was introduced in 1980, the UK chose a support system which involved a ewe premium and a premium based on the final product, the slaughter lamb.

The basis of the UK system is as follows:

(1) A weekly guaranteed price ('Guide-price') is agreed:

(a) Set annually for Great Britain by the Council of Ministers.

(b) Seasonal changes over the year are marked and thus influence farmers' marketing policy. The pattern of seasonal changes was changed in 1984 so that prices fell steeply during June and July. This meant that if farmers do not get lambs to slaughter weight by July, there was little commercial incentive to send them for slaughter until November, since the guide price remains the same throughout August and September.

e.g. In 1989, the lowest guide-price was 203p/kg estimated dressed carcase weight (edcw = half live weight) and the highest was 252 p/kg.

The'best' live weight at which to market lambs of different breeds and crosses can be estimated as follows:

live weight = (sum of weight of mature ram and ewe) / 4

This does not remove the necessity to handle individual lambs but gives an indication of the best weight at which to slaughter in order to produce a lean carcase.

(2) The average UK market price is frequently lower than the guide price. eg. in January 1989, the guide price was 245p/kg and the market price was 144p/kg.

(3) Difference between guide price and average market price is made up by the payment of a 'variable premium' to producers, from EEC funds. e.g. in January 1989, the variable premium was 101p/kg, which was exceptionally high. Over 1988, the variable premium averaged 58.8p/kg out of a total return of 235.8p/kg (25%).

This premium is only paid on 'certified' carcases and it is essential that all carcases should be certified for a farmer to be successful.

(4) The certification system is operated by MLC graders and discourages fat carcases. The carcase classification method uses a grid whereby a value is given for degree of fatness and another value for conformation. Fat classes run from 1 to 5 in increasing fatness, with 3 and 4 subdivided into L and H. Conformation classes are E, U, R, O and P in decreasing conformation. A carcase is described as U3L, for example. Carcases which are over fat (4H) and of poor conformation (P) are rejected for variable premium but, in addition, many abattoirs will pay a higher price for carcases of a certain classification. Farmers should aim for a carcase which is at least as good as R3L, which number only around 50% of lambs sold at present.

(5) Exporters to EEC countries (France being most important for UK) have to pay a levy, which is equal to the variable premium – this is the so-called 'claw-back'. The 'claw-back' is not payable on exports to non-EEC countries.

(6) In addition to 'variable premium', which is paid on the final product, two types of ewe premiums are paid

(a) Annual ewe premium paid entirely from EEC funds. This is paid on all ewes and depends on the annual average market price of lamb. A calculation is made in retrospect to bring the average producer's return up to a 'Reference Price' which is agreed by the Ministers at the beginning of the marketing year in April. The emphasis has been for the ewe premium to increase over the 5 years of the regime and the average ewe premium is now about £6.00.

(b) Less Favoured Areas premium.The EEC recognises that certain areas (especially hill areas) are particularly difficult to farm, production costs being high and farm incomes below non-agricultural incomes. Member countries may pay a compensatory allowance to such farmers, limits being set for its amount, 25% of its cost coming from EEC funds and 75% from the member country. The annual compensatory allowances in Britain are £6.75 for specified breeds and £4.50 for other breeds on hills and £2.25 for upland ewes.

The variable premium scheme outlined in the foregoing does not apply to Northern Ireland in order that its scheme agrees with that obtaining in Eire where the payments are entirely on the ewe premium basis.

Examples of MLC Records (figures from the 1988 lambing season)
Variable costs are those which can be assigned to the sheep section on a mixed farm and vary with the number of sheep kept. These are used in the calculation of gross margin.
The average results are quoted with the results for the 'top-third' of flocks in brackets.
Fixed costs must be deducted to obtain net margin, i.e. gross margin less labour, rent, depreciation; these vary considerably between different enterprises.

HILL (based on 25 flocks – a very small number, so is not representative)

Physical results (per 100 ewes to tup)		
Lambs born	116	(123)
Lambs reared	109	(118)
% lambs sold direct to slaughter	26	(19)
% lambs retained for breeding	36	(42)
Barren ewes	6	(4)
Dead ewes	2	(1)
Productive ewes	93	(95)

Income (per ewe to ram) £			Variable costs £		
Sale of lambs/valuation	24.59	(32.85)	Ewe concentrates	3.28	(3.91)
Sale of draft ewes	7.10	(8.06)	Other purchased feed	3.75	(4.22)
Wool	1.80	(1.92)	Forage/grassland costs	2.36	(2.32)
Premium and subsidy	13.17	(13.12)	Vet/medicines	2.37	(2.83)
			Market/transport etc	0.65	(0.53)
Gross returns	46.66	(55.95)	Total	9.13	(9.90)
Less flock replacements (rams)	2.04	(1.49)			
Output	44.62	(54.46)	Gross margin per ewe	35.49	(44.56)

UPLAND (130 flocks, selling lambs for slaughter and as stores)

Physical results (per 100 ewes to tup)		
Lambs born	149	(151)
Lambs reared	136	(136)
% lambs sold direct to slaughter	48	(53)
% lambs retained for breeding	13	(13)
Barren ewes	6	(7)
Dead ewes	2	(2)
Productive ewes	92	(91)

Income (per ewe to ram) £			Variable costs £		
Sale of lambs/valuation	50.78	(51.85)	Ewe concentrates	5.65	(5.27)
Wool	2.59	(2.61)	Other purchased feed	0.44	(0.38)
Premium and subsidy	10.04	(10.04)	Forage/grassland costs	4.85	(4.53)
			Vet/medicines	3.00	(2.73)
			Market/transport etc	1.14	(0.99)
Gross returns	63.41	(64.50)	Total	15.08	(13.90)
Less flock replacements (rams)	8.38	(4.92)			
Output	55.03	(59.58)	Gross margin per ewe	39.95	(45.68)
			Gross margin per ha	419	(640)

LOWLAND (407 flocks, selling lambs for slaughter and as stores)

Physical results (per 100 ewes to tup)		
Lambs born	168	(181)
Lambs reared	151	(156)
% lambs sold direct to slaughter	47	(52)
% lambs retained for breeding	6	(6)
Barren ewes	6	(6)
Dead ewes	5	(5)
Productive ewes	92	(92)

Income (per ewe to ram) £			Variable costs £		
Sale of lambs/valuation	57.16	(60.39)	Ewe concentrates	7.54	(6.57)
Wool	3.05	(3.12)	Other purchased feed	2.32	(2.37)
Premium	6.05	(6.38)	Forage/grassland costs	5.03	(4.77)
			Vet/medicines	3.85	(3.58)
			Market/transport etc	1.58	(1.45)
Gross returns	66.26	(69.89)	Total	20.32	(18.74)
Less flock replacements (rams)	9.89	(7.71)			
Output	56.37	(62.12)	Gross margin per ewe	36.05	(43.38)
Stocking rate (grass and forage)					
ewes per ha	12.8	(15.60)			
Kg nitrogen per ha	157	(177)	Gross margin per ha	461	(677)

(7) In order to limit the amount of financial support to the sheep industry, a system of 'stabilisers' was introduced in May 1988. For the UK, a standard population of 18.1 million ewes is assumed and every 1% increase in ewe number leads to a 1% reduction in support prices. Increased ewe numbers in UK have already led to a reduction of 7% in support price by January 1989.

(8) More fundamental changes in the Regime are under discussion with a view to complete introduction by 1992, the year of the Single Market, including the phasing-out of the variable premium, a limit on the payment of ewe premiums to 500 ewes on lowland farms and 1000 ewes on hill farms and payments for reducing ewe stocking rates as part of an'extensification' campaign. These measures would profoundly alter marketing and agricultural practices and are the subject of complex forecasts by MLC and the National Sheep Association (see publications).

Further reading:
MLC publications, especially *Market Outlook* and *Sheep Yearbook*.
National Sheep Association, *The Sheep Farmer* (published monthly).

CONTROL OF BREEDING

There are now a considerable number of methods which advance the breeding season or synchronise tupping and lambing.

(1) Early lambing with progestagen sponges

Discuss with the farmer when he can sell finished lambs, and whether he wants lambs born before Christmas or after. (Pedigree ram lambs should be born after 1 January.)

e.g. calculate: last lambing	23 December
if longest gestation 150 days, remove rams	26 July
if rams with ewes 3 and 4 days after sponges out, remove sponges	22 July
if sponges in for 13 days, insert sponges	9 July

Veramix Sheep Sponges (Upjohn Ltd) contain 60mg medroxyprogesterone acetate. Veramix Plus (Upjohn Ltd) are similar but supplied with pregnant mares serum gonadotrophin (PMSG). Chronogest (Intervet UK Ltd) contains 30mg fluorogestone acetate.

Roughly 70% of the ewes should lamb to the induced oestrus and most have twins. Results vary widely, according to breed, feeding, time of year and weather. Test a batch of ewes and record the results in order to find out whether the procedure is worthwhile on a particular farm. Recommended dose of PMSG ranges from 300 – 600 i.u. at sponge withdrawal, with a higher dose in July than in August. Ewes and rams should be in good condition (Score 3) and fit. If possible, remove ewes from the ram when they have been marked (raddled) convincingly,to avoid repeated serving of favourites. Put the rams near the ewes at sponge withdrawal, and put them with the ewes 48 hours after withdrawal, for 48 hours. Introducing rams at sponge withdrawal reduces the pregnancy rate drastically (68% to 40% in one trial). Two weeks after first oestrus, put rams with the ewes for one week, with different raddle crayon, and then remove. The usual advice is to allow 1 ram for 10 ewes, though it is possible with some individual rams to achieve good fertility with more ewes. There are big differences between individuals and between breeds in the ability of rams to breed outside the usual season.

Only well-managed farms can benefit from early, concentrated lambings. Marketing of lambs, and housing and labour for lambings must be planned well. MLC figures for 1987 show a higher gross margin from early lambs (£530/hectare) than from grass lambs (£437/hectare), brought about by a much higher stocking rate in the early lambing flocks, due to the absence of lambs during the grazing season.

In theory, ewes may be weaned early, mated in February without hormone help, and three crops of lambs produced every two years. In practice, very few people have achieved this. Dr W M Tempest, of Harper Adams Agricultural College, has managed a successful system which produces lambs every 8 months from ewes mated in December, April and August. He uses Finnish Landrace X Dorset Horn ewes and Down rams. Lamb sales approaching 300% and profitability three times higher than in annual lambing flocks are reported. We are aware of one other commercial farm where this is carried out successfully.

(2) Early breeding with vasectomised rams

A vasectomised ram run with ewes one to two months earlier than the usual start of the breeding season will stimulate a large proportion of the flock to come into oestrus about 3–4 weeks after his introduction. The ewes must be away from rams for 4 – 6 weeks before the teaser is introduced. This is a cheap method of inducing synchronised oestrus. The vasectomised ram may also be used to withdraw individual ewes, as they are raddled, for service by a fertile ram, or for artificial insemination.

(3) Effect of shearing on start of breeding season

Clun ewes which were shorn before mid July began to cycle earlier than ewes which were not shorn until early August. (During the same period in different years a higher mean ambient temperature delayed the onset of breeding: a difference of 2.1°C (3.8°F) was associated with a difference of 20 days.)

(4) Out of season breeding with progestagen sponges and PMSG

Disappointing results have been obtained earlier than July. A successful attempt was made by Liverpool University in 40 barren or aborted cross-bred ewes in North Wales. Sponges were removed and 1000 units PMSG injected on 25 May. Twenty ewes lambed, producing 30 live and 7 dead lambs, and the lambs fetched a high price when sold for slaughter.

Elvidge from Oxford University has mated Mule (Blue-faced Leicester X Swaledale) ewes in June, with progestagen sponges and PMSG (Veramix Plus, Upjohn Ltd), with 50% of ewes becoming pregnant.

(5) Out of season breeding with light control

Sheep that are housed may be given a shortening day-length, to induce cycling.

(6) Melatonin

If melatonin is fed at 3 – 5pm, the sheep behaves as if the night is longer. A ruminal glass bolus or intravaginal coil containing melatonin has a similar effect. The ewes lamb earlier, over a shorter period and with a higher lambing percentage, since ovulation rate is higher in the middle of the breeding season.

(7) Batch lambing during the breeding season

Progestagen sponges (without PMSG) may be used. Prostaglandins may also be used but fertility in the induced oestrus has been poorer than after sponges. The second oestrus is well synchronised. Two doses are given 10 days apart. Cloprostenol (Estrumate, Coopers Pitman-Moore,100 μg) or dinoprost (Lutalyse, Upjohn Ltd, 15 mg) are effective.

(8) Induction of lambing

Predictable lambing dates can be achieved by injecting 8ml (16mg) betamethasone or dexamethasone 140 days of gestation or later.

In a trial in 1983 at Liverpool University, 33 ewes were selected for injection with betamethasone (Betsolan Injection, Coopers Pitman-Moore, 16 mg) at 9pm on day 142 of pregnancy (Saturday). Two lambed before treatment, 3 within 24 hours, 3 between 24 and 36 hours, and 24 between 36 and 48 hours (9am–9pm Monday). Only one ewe lambed later, 55 hours after treatment. It is clearly possible to give better attention to ewes, and to give attendants a rest, particularly avoiding the few ewes at the end of a group with long gestations. Side-effects appear to be negligible, but if some ewes have been mated after the recorded service date (e.g. one cycle later), there is a serious risk of abortion.

(9) Increasing lambing percentage by immunisation

Immunisation against androstenedione (Fecundin Injection, Coopers Pitman-Moore) increases the ovulation rate, by preventing the physiological inhibition of gonadotrophin. A 2ml dose is given 8 and 4 weeks before tupping begins. In subsequent years, one dose is given 4 weeks before tupping. One ml contains 0.6mg ovandrotone albumin.

An ADAS trial showed 23 extra lambs from every 100 ewes tupped. They advise using it on flocks with lambing rates between 120 and 160%. In one farm, Scottish Blackface ewes on a hill showed no response, whereas ewes on improved pasture produced 12% more lambs. To cover the costs, about 10% more lambs are needed. It is important that adequate nutrition, shelter and supervision should be given to the ewes or the increased lamb numbers born will be offset by increased lamb mortality. The effect of lifetime profitability needs to be assessed.

Ram Examination

This is best done 2 months before tupping time and at flock health visits. About 10% of rams have poor fertility. Many of these can be detected by palpation of testicles, and most by examination of fresh semen.

Examination of a ram lamb before use, or of a freshly-bought ram, is a wise investment. An infertile ram which is not detected can lead to ewes lambing two months late. If several rams of the same breed work together, an infertile ram may never be detected and may result in a reduction in overall fertility of the flock.

Any history based on good breeding records is valuable. Illness, however brief, can lead to temporary or permanent infertility up to two months later. If the ram is examined before entry to the flock, his conformation and any inherited condition should be checked. Teeth should make contact with the dental pad. Orf should be looked for around the lips. Condition score should be 3 to 3.5. Feet should be checked; about 50% of rams were found to have severe foot lesions in one survey, which can drastically reduce fertility.

Before the breeding season (before July in the British Isles), the size of testicles and numbers of spermatozoa are lower, especially in breeds with a short season.

The testicles should be of similar size, very firm (turgid) and move freely in the scrotum (compare with others of the same age and similar breed). The scrotal circumference ranges from 30–44cm in mature lowland rams and from 30–40 cm in hill breeds. Ram lambs at 9 months old should be at least 28cm in lowland, 26cm in hill breeds. Testicular hypoplasia is incurable: no spermatozoa are produced, though libido is normal.

The penis can be extended with care in the sitting position, to check for rare defects, by holding the prepuce and pushing forwards with the other hand at the sigmoid flexure, which is found at the base of the testicles.

Electroejaculators can be powered by mains electricity (Semen Sampler, Centaur Veterinary Equipment, Edinburgh) or by battery (Ruakura type, Alfred Cox).The tip of the probe should be on the pubic brim, but there are marks to indicate the depth of insertion in the average ram's rectum. The method has been criticised on welfare grounds and it seems preferable to avoid electroejaculation unless there are strong grounds for suspecting the ram is infertile. In addition, it seems reasonable to give up if a sample is not obtained after 3 or 4 attempts and try again later. The ram can stand or lie. The semen can be collected in a warm beaker or into a small transparent plastic bag. Between 0.5 and 2ml of dense creamy semen is normally collected from a fertile ram. Semen obtained by electroejaculation is not necessarily typical of a natural ejaculate and some breed societies require examination by artificial vagina, which often needs training (for the ram!).

Semen examined immediately on a warm slide in a warm room should show good wave motion (as if being vigorously stirred) as seen in bull semen. If a poor sample is obtained, a second sample should normally be taken. After mixing one drop of semen on a warm slide with 5 drops of nigrosin-eosin (1.67g eosin, 10.0g nigrosin, 100ml water) for three minutes, a smear can be made. The total number, number live (unstained), and number free of morphological abnormalities provide further evidence of the likely fertility.

If the history and examination of the ram and semen show reduced fertility, treatment is not normally possible. A potentially valuable ram may be tested again two months later, as infertility is occasionally temporary. A report should always remind the client that the only final evidence of fertility is the production of lambs.

Artificial Insemination (AI)

AI in British sheep is not yet common. In 1984 the Meat and Livestock Commission (MLC) for the first time offered a commercial insemination service to 1000 ewes within 50 miles of their Pig Breeding Centre, Thorpe Willoughby, Selby. Fresh semen pooled from Suffolk rams selected for fast growth gave a non-return rate (NRR) of 71%.

The advantages for a market where little premium is paid on quality is in fast growth of lambs.

The cost, including synchronisation by intravaginal sponge, and 500 iu PMSG at withdrawal, is about £5. Withdrawal at 8 am is followed by AI at 4pm 2 days later (56 hours). Clearly, pooled semen is inappropriate for pedigree breeders, who can, however, obtain advice and help from MLC, including training in collection and insemination.

Fresh semen can be placed in the vagina or preferably, by pipette, just into the cervix, allowing one ejaculate to inseminate 10–20 ewes with a conception rate of about 70%. Unfortunately, conception rates with frozen semen placed into the cervix are low (30%) even if the dose of sperm is increased to 400×10^6, which would allow only about 5 ewes to be inseminated from one ejaculate. Much better results (70% conception rate) have been obtained by intrauterine insemination by laparoscopy, under local analgesia, with a dose as low as 20×10^6, which means that about 100 ewes can be inseminated from one ejaculate.

Although questions have been raised about the ethics of this procedure and of the collection of eggs from the uterus after superovulation for embryo transfer by laparoscopy (Multiple Ovulation Embryo Transfer -MOET), the stress to the ewe from a 5mm laparoscope appears to be small. Commercial companies are offering both AI and MOET by laparoscopy to sheep breeders.

Reference Sires

The Scottish Agricultural Colleges have recently introduced a scheme for selecting rams objectively for traits measured in a variety of environments.

Previously, rams were chosen subjectively from pedigree flocks. Only weight achieved from the nominal starting date of 1 January could be measured.

AI with frozen semen allows a ram to be tested in many flocks at the same time. Ultrasonic measurement of depth of fat and of muscle provides objective measurement of carcase quality in live lambs.

Lambs from several rams are, therefore, bred in several flocks. The analysis is said to be complex, since the lambs are half-sibs, and in different farms.

Costs are estimated at £16 per ewe for AI, £20 per ewe for semen, and £2 per lamb for scanning. Alternatives include a central ram-testing station which would be expensive and a potential risk to health.

Further reading
Meat and Livestock Commission Yearbook, 1989

Group Breeding Scheme

In the last 10 years, several groups of breeders in the UK have used experience in New Zealand to establish schemes.

A group breeding scheme uses a nucleus flock to which the best ewes from the base flocks are transferred, and which supplies rams to the base flocks. Ten to twelve members each pay towards running the nucleus. Schemes exist for Welsh Mountain, Lleyn, Romney, Beulah and Texel breeds.

A few schemes are based on several cooperating recorded flocks, called an open nucleus.

Diagnosis of Pregnancy and Number of Lambs by Ultrasonic Scanning

A large number of people have now set up as scanners, and an organisation called Ewescan exists to ensure quality control among affiliated users (Newton Bank, Frankscroft, Peebles). For 50p to £1 a ewe, the number of foetuses is estimated, with errors less than 2% for experienced operators, and some 2 million ewes have been scanned annually in the past few years. An experienced operator can scan 80-120 ewes per hour.

The value of the technique is that barren ewes can be sold when prices are high, or fed less until later, ewes with single lambs can be fed less, saving feed, and avoiding over-large lambs, and ewes with two or more lambs can be fed more concentrates and watched carefully for loss of condition or pregnancy toxaemia. The Hill Farming Research Organisation (HFRO) and ADAS have estimated the value of scanning at £3.00 – £4.50 a ewe, but the major contribution to this saving is an estimate of the reduced mortality rate of the lambs. If lamb mortality is already low and if lambing % is near to 200, the economic advantages are much less.

The original machines used a linear array and, for this, the ewes must be shorn to 20cm cranial to the udder, across the whole ventral abdomen, and kept off roughage for 8 hours. They either lie in a cradle or sit up. Recent machines have a sector array and may be used with the ewes in the standing position without shearing. For accurate diagnosis of foetal numbers, the flock should be scanned between 80 and 105 days after the beginning of mating, allowing a 35 day period with tups in the flock.

Other methods of diagnosing foetal numbers include X-ray (more expensive, not generally available, slightly hazardous), measurement of progesterone in blood (unreliable) and Doppler ultrasound (unreliable).

The main alternative is regular condition scoring and transfer of thin ewes to groups fed more concentrates. This avoids the need for pregnancy diagnosis, but requires regular examination by good shepherds during late pregnancy.

Further reading

Henderson, D (1985). 'Control of the breeding season in sheep and goats' *In Practice*, Vol. 7, 118–23.

Logue, D and Greig, A. 'Infertility in the bull, ram and boar' *In Practice*, (1985), Vol. 7, 185–91; (1986), Vol. 8, 118–22; (1987), Vol. 9, 167–70.

Haresign, W (1987). 'The use of laparoscopy as an aid to artificial insemination and embryo transfer in sheep', *Proceedings of the Sheep Veterinary Society*, Vol. 12, 96–102.

FEEDING MANAGEMENT

Grass, either fresh or conserved, is the main feedstuff for sheep in the United Kingdom. However, because of seasonal effects and varying requirements during the production cycle, there are periods during the year when grass needs to be supplemented with concentrates.

Feeding the Ram

Rams must be in fit condition 6 – 8 weeks before mating with a condition score of 3 to 4. In many circumstances, this will be achieved by providing reasonable grazing. If grass is insufficient then concentrates may need to be fed in the two month period prior to and during the mating season. Up to 400g/day of a 16g/100g (16%) crude protein concentrate is advised, but overfeeding should be avoided. Frequently, rams are neglected and are in poor condition not only because of inadequate feeding but also because of parasites, bad feet and other health problems.

Feeding the Ewe

There are three important periods when grass supplies may need to be supplemented.

(1) Pre- and immediate post-mating

(2) Late pregnancy.

(3) Early lactation.

(1) Pre- and immediate post-mating

Ewes in below optimum condition at this stage will have lower ovulation and conception rates and increased likelihood of barrenness. The optimum condition score for hill and mountain ewes is 3.0 and for lowland ewes 3.5, with within flock ranges of 2.5 - 3.5 and 3.0 - 4.0, respectively. Ideally, ewes should gain weight in the pre-mating period, be in good condition at mating and remain so for a month post-mating.

Adequate amounts of grass of reasonable quality must therefore be provided for two months in the late summer and autumn, which necessitates the farmer reserving an area of pasture for this purpose. In some situations, more especially in later lambing flocks, grass may have to be supplemented with concentrates; the actual amounts fed will, however, vary considerably and will be dependent on grass availability and ewe condition. Poor condition ewes need careful investigation – the presence of significant numbers is usually associated with underfeeding and overstocking. However, poor condition may also be attributable to health problems such as faulty teeth or fascioliasis.

(2) Late pregnancy - 8/6 weeks pre-partum

This coincides, in most cases, with winter months when grass is of inferior quality and there is little available. Conserved forage is therefore the main source of nutrients with concentrates provided when necessary.

The amount of concentrates to feed depends on:

(a) Quantity of forage available

(b) Quality of forage available (any grass available will be equivalent to medium or poor quality hay).

The quality of conserved grass will be determined by the dry matter content (DM) in the case of silage and in both hay and silage by the digestibility of the organic matter in the dry matter ('D' value), by the metabolisable energy concentration (ME) and by the crude protein content (CP). These may be obtained directly or indirectly by chemical analysis of the foodstuff (see later). A good guide on the farm can be obtained by assessment of the stage of maturity when the grass was conserved, and, for silage, by estimating the dry matter percentage (squeeze) and type of fermentation (smell). Grass cut early will be leafy, have few seed heads and will produce high quality forage; on the other hand, if cutting is delayed far beyond the emergence of the inflorescence, poor quality material will result consisting mainly of seed heads and stalky lignified stems.

(c) Live weight of the ewe.

(d) Condition of the ewe.

Scoring at 8 – 6 weeks pre-lambing, which may coincide with housing, and 4–2 weeks pre-partum, when vaccinating for clostridial disease, will provide a good guide to the adequacy of feeding. Lowland ewes should have a condition score of 3.5, upland or mountain ewes 2.5 or more at both times. If ewes have been sheared, changes in condition score can be easily observed.

(e) Foetal load.

This can be estimated on the basis of previous performances of the flock, and the estimate may have to be modified in individual cases in the last weeks of pregnancy if the condition score changes rapidly. Ultra-sound scanning by trained operators gives an accurate prediction of the number of lambs being carried.

(f) Stage of pregnancy.

The use of ram raddles at mating time gives extra precision to gestation time.

(g) Appetite level.

Dry matter intake is approximately 1.5% of live weight in early and mid pregnancy but increases in the latter stages to 2.0 – 2.5% until the last few days, when there is a marked decline.

There is, however, considerable variability; the digestibility of the ration will have a major influence with poor quality, high fibre diets causing physical restriction and reduced appetite.

Predicting appetite level for a range of diets is difficult and is one of the main problems of ration formulation.

Steps in the construction of a suitable ration for a 70kg ewe of condition score 3.5 carrying twins from 8 weeks pre-partum

(i) Obtain an estimate of the quantity and quality of foods available

Compositional quality of some common foodstuffs figures are on oven-dry basis for ME, protein and mineral levels.

	DM (g/100g)	ME (MJ/kg)	CP (g/100g)	CP degradability	Ca (g/100g)	P (g/100g)	Mg (g/100g)
Hay							
medium quality	86	8.7	9.0	0.8	0.3	0.2	0.08
good quality	86	9.5	11.0	0.8	0.3	0.3	0.16
Silage	25	10.5	14.5	0.8	0.3	0.3	0.16
Concentrates							
oats	87	12.5	10.0	0.8	0.08	0.35	0.1
barley	87	13.0	9.5	0.8	0.06	0.4	0.1
soya bean meal	90	12.2	45.0	0.6	0.3	0.75	0.3
fish meal	90	11.0	63.0	0.3	6.0	3.8	0.2

Typical mineral/vitamin mix composition (g/100g): Ca = 15, P = 8, Mg = 12, NaC1 = 15; and (ppm): Mn = 4000, Fe = 3000, Zn = 1000, I_2 = 40, Co= 20, Se = 10; and (iu/g): Vit A = 400, Vit D_3 = 40, Vit E = 0.8.

Note that:

(a) The most variable feedstuffs are the forages and there could be some value in having hay and silage samples analysed chemically. The ME concentration can be calculated from the fibre level in the foodstuff by the following formula:

Hay ME (MJ/kg DM) = 16.5 – 0.21 x Modified Acid Detergent (MAD) fibre.

*Silage ME (MJ/kg DM) = D x 0.186 x DM $^{-0.0294}$ where D = Organic Matter (OM) (0.1 – 0.00009225 x MAD fibre). D is expressed as a % and OM and MAD fibre as g/kg DM.

The ME value can also be predicted directly from 'D' values by the equation ME = 0.15 D.

(b) The crude protein content can also be obtained by analysis. However, the figure obtained may be inflated because the analysis and calculation assumes all the nitrogen measured has a protein source.

(c) Compound foods may also vary. The ME value of such foods can be predicted from the declared analysis by the following equation:

[+] ME = 12.0 + 0.08CP + 0.23 EE – 0.18 CF – 0.12 TA or [++]ME = 0.25 EE + 0.14 NCD

CP = crude protein, EE = ether extract, CF = crude fibre, TA = total ash, NCD = neutral cellulase digestibility.

(All analytical values are expressed as percentages in the dry matter.)

(d) The degradability of the protein is a measure of the proportion likely to be degraded

*Source: AFRC (1987), *Nutrition Abstracts and Reviews (Series B)*, No. 9, Vol. 57, 507–23.
[+]Source: MAFF Reference Book 433, *Energy allowances and feeding systems for ruminants.*
[++]Source: Thomas, P.C., 50th Easter School in Agricultural Science, University of Nottingham.

in the rumen (rumen degradable protein [RDP]), and how much will escape microbial action and pass directly into the abomasum (undegradable protein [UDP]).

(e) In some cases, the source of protein and minerals and vitamins will be a 'supermix' product. This is often more convenient for the farmer but the information of the mineral/vitamin levels for specific ingredients is not often readily available. A straight mineral/vitamin mix will usually have such a detailed analysis. The analysis varies from product to product so it should be possible to choose one which will meet specific needs. It should be remembered that consumption depends not only on the inclusion rate but also on the amounts being fed.

(ii) Estimate ewe requirements and appetite per day

Weeks pre-partum		8	6	4	2	0
Appetite						
dry matter (oven dry)	(kg)	1.3	1.35	1.5	1.65	1.3
Requirements						
ME	(MJ)	11	13	15	17.5	20.5
crude protein	(g)	110	140	155	180	290
degradability		0.8	0.8	0.8	0.75	0.55
Ca	(g)	4	6	6.6	7	8
P	(g)	2	3	4	4	5
Mg	(g)	1.5	1.5	1.7	1.7	2.0
NaC1	(g)	2.0	2.0	2.5	2.5	3.0

Note that:

(a) Maintenance

ME = 0.42 MJ/kg wt $^{0.75}$

Nett protein = 2.4g/kg wt $^{0.75}$

Production	@ days of gestation 102	116	130	144
ME (MJ/kg lamb birthweight)	0.37	0.55	0.73	0.90
Nett protein (g/MJ ME for production)	5.3	5.3	6.1	11.7

RDP and UDP levels can be calculated from the nett protein figures.

Nett protein from degradable source = ME intake (MJ) x 4.35

Crude protein from degradable source

= ME (MJ) x 4.35 x 0.544 (absorption x digestion x rumen loss proportions)

Crude protein from undegradable source

= Nett protein - nett protein from degradable source x 0.68

(0.68 = absorption x digestion proportions)

(b) The above figures have to be adjusted when ewes of different weight and condition scores are being considered and when ewes have a higher foetal load. The approximate adjustments suggested are a 10% change for a difference of 10kg live weight or 1 unit of condition score, and a 20% increase for ewes carrying triplets.

(iii) Calculate amounts to feed (g DM/day)

e.g. with the following available foods- moderate quality hay, barley, soya bean meal, fish meal and sheep mineral mix .

Weeks pre-partum	8 to 6	6 to 4	4 to 2	2 to 0
Hay	1290	1080	900	470
Concentrates				
barley	-	280	620	980
soya bean meal	-	43	35	90
fish meal	-	-	-	80
vit/min mix	-	25	25	25
Total	-	348	680	1175

Note that:

(a) The amounts shown above are for oven dry materials. It is necessary, therefore, to include a factor for DM% in the calculations, eg. @ 8 weeks an intake of 1.3kg oven dry hay is equivalent to 1.3 x 100/86 = 1.5kg air dry material weighed on the farm.

(b) As much forage as possible is included to minimise costs. Hay levels are approximate and reflect appetite; it is important to establish that the animals are actually eating these amounts, especially with poor quality material with which wastage can be considerable.

(c) The allowances are given for 2 week periods and are based on the mean nutrient requirement for this time span. In certain circumstances, weekly adjustments may be necessary but are generally of little benefit. Flat rate feeding concentrates is an extreme modification to the steadily increasing rationing system outlined above. This system involves calculating the total concentrate need for a particular period, which may even be the 8 weeks pre-partum, and then dividing into equal daily aliquots for the whole period which makes daily feeding easier. As a result, ewes increase in weight and condition in the early part of each period and lose considerable amounts in the later stages. The full effects of this can be reduced to some extent by changing the quality of roughage fed which should be available ad libitum.

(d) In the last days of pregnancy, requirements are not being met so the ewe will lose condition. Feeding higher quality hay would improve the situation, but increasing the concentrate intake could cause metabolic upsets (cereal over-eating). Feeding whole barley reduces the risk of this occurring, as does the feeding of a complete diet. Deficits in nutrient intake at this time are offset by the mobilisation of the body reserves of the ewe. It is recommended that reserves are built up prior to the final week of pregnancy by providing more nutrients than is theoretically required. This is especially important in the case of protein, for which there is a high requirement for udder development and colostrum production in the last days of pregnancy.

(e) Pregnancy toxaemia may occur if only good quality forage is provided. This is because, although total energy is sufficient, there is a lack of glucose energy which is normally synthesised from propionic acid. Including a supply of readily digestible carbohydrates overcomes the problem.

(f) The consequences of under-nutrition are smaller lambs with higher mortality, reduced colostrum and milk yield and increased body condition loss and incidence of pregnancy toxaemia. The farmer, however, may accept lower performance if this means substantial cost saving; in particular, the protein level may be deliberately kept below the above. Economies made at this stage can have long-lasting effects and are usually ill-advised.

(3) Early Lactation

The same principles of ration formulation apply. Spring grass is, however, often available to meet part or all of the ewe's needs.

Requirements and appetite level per day for 70kg ewe of CS 3.5 suckling twins each growing @ 300g/day:

Weeks post-partum		1	2	4	6	8
Approximate milk yield (litres)		2.5	3.0	3.2	3.0	2.5
Appetite DM (kg)						
concentrates + hay		2.0	2.4	2.6	2.6	2.4
grass only		2.5	2.8	3.0	3.0	2.8
Requirements						
ME	(MJ)	28	32	34	32	28
RDP	(g)	185	240	240	232	225
UDP	(g)	114	105	120	112	82
Total CP	(g)	300	345	360	344	307
Ca	(g)	12	14	14	14	12
Mg	(g)	3.5	4.0	4.5	4.0	3.0
P	(g)	9	10	10	10	9
NaCl	(g)	5	6	6	6	5

Note that:

(a) The following equations have been used to compile the requirements:

(i) ME

Maintenance = 0.42 MJ/$wt^{0.75}$

Production = 4.5 MJ/kg milk

(ii) Nett protein

Maintenance = 2.4 g/$wt^{0.75}$

Production = 48 g/kg milk

RDP and UDP have been calculated as indicated above.

(b) The milk yield of ewes may be estimated by assuming that the dry matter percentage of ewes' milk is 20% and the food conversion ratio of dry matter of milk to live weight gain is 1:1. In the situation specified above the estimated milk yield is therefore 2 x 300 = 600 x 5 = 3.0 litres/day.

(c) Appetite increases up to the 5th or 6th week of lactation, although milk yield peaks at the 3rd or 4th week.

Amounts to feed (g/day)

Weeks post-partum	1	2	4	6	8
Hay (good quality)	600	700	800	800	700
Concentrates					
barley	1150	1450	1510	1510	1410
soya bean meal	180	210	250	250	250
fish meal	40	40	10	10	-
vit/min mix	30	30	30	30	30
Total	1400	1730	1800	1800	1690
Body weight change	-	-	-	=	+

Note that:

(a) In early lactation, it is not possible to meet the theoretical requirements so some loss in body condition will occur. Provided ewes are in condition score 3 or better (lowland ewes) or 2.5 or better (hill), a loss of 1 condition score is unlikely to affect milk yield. Protein levels have been adjusted for likely body weight changes of the ewe.

(b) When little or no grass is available, it is necessary to feed good quality hay in the first month of lactation, together with a concentrate containing fish meal or some other source of undegradable protein.

(c) Alternative forages, e.g. silage or straw, and alternative concentrates, e.g. sugar beet pulp, maize gluten, oats, grass meal, may be used.

(d) Feeding conserved forage and concentrates alone is unusual after 4 weeks of lactation in flocks lambing from late February onwards.

(e) If grass is available at any time, the concentrate and hay rations can be reduced. At grass, if there is an insufficient supply, supplementation with a concentrate including fish meal has a beneficial effect on milk yield and lamb growth. Providing cereals alone results only in reduction in ewe weight loss. However, at grass, provision should be made for ewes to receive magnesium in early lactation; up to 6g calcined magnesite is recommended. If abundant grass is available, the theoretical requirement can be met without supplementation.

Feeding the Lamb

The ewe should supply sufficient milk for twin lambs to survive and grow well. Milk is the only source of nutrients to 3 weeks of age and the main supplier to 8 weeks. From week 4 onwards, the lamb will eat measurable quantities of grass and/or creep feed concentrate if milk is not in abundant supply, e.g. in the case of triplet lambs reared on the ewe.

Most pre-lambing mortality occurs in the first few days of life and the major cause is starvation. Insufficient milk may be due to the ewe not allowing the lamb to suck or to a lack of supply due to poor nutrition during pregnancy or to udder problems. Starvation after the first few days is usually the result of poor feeding of the ewe in lactation or of sore teats or mastitis.

Providing the lamb with a supply of colostrum is essential. Ideally, the lamb will receive this from its dam within a few hours of birth and will continue to suck its dam and receive further amounts in the following 48 hours. Lambs will consume more than 1000ml in the first day but 100-200ml is considered enough to give disease protection provided the colostrum is from the first two withdrawals of milk. If lambs are weak or slow, it may be given via a stomach tube.

Lack of supply may be overcome by collecting surplus colostrum from ewes and deep freezing until required. Alternatively, cow colostrum can be used; however, this will have no clostridial antibodies unless the cow has been previously vaccinated. Vaccination should be done at 3 months, 1 month and 2 weeks pre-calving. It is essential that the milk from the first two withdrawals is collected. It can then be deep frozen in aliquots of 200ml. The value of colostrum to the lamb declines after 1 day of age, but there will be some absorption of immunoglobulin after this time, especially if the lamb has been partially starved in the first 24 hours of life.

After 2 days, lambs which are surplus to the ewe's rearing capacity can be reared artificially. The following is an outline of an efficient and economic way of accomplishing this:

Day 2:

Introduce milk replacer. It is best to have a product with 30% fat in the powder and to mix it in the ratio by weight of 1:4 with either warm or cold water. Initially, lambs take more readily to warm milk, but it is possible to use either a warm milk restricted feed 3 feeds per day system or to feed milk ad libitum. Intakes in the latter system will reach 2.5 to 3.0 litres, whilst on restricted feed 1.5 litres per day is considered the maximum to feed. Lambs on restricted intake can be fed with a bucket with teats at the base, but when feeding is ad libitum, the teats need to be above milk level with a polythene tube into the milk. A food conversion of 1:1, i.e. 1kg milk powder producing 1kg live weight gain, can be expected.

Day 14:

Introduce solid food and feed ad libitum. Alternative diets are whole barley plus a protein mineral balancer or a pelleted complete diet of the following composition (g/100g): coarsely milled straw, 15, barley, 70, and good sources of UDP such as soya bean and fish meal to give a 16 g/100g (oven dry) crude protein level. A source of long fibre should also be made available to help stimulate early food consumption. This can be fed ad libitum throughout the growing and finishing periods without adverse effects on performance. The mineral content should be sufficient to provide for healthy growth but should include little or none of a mineral source of phosphorus or magnesium to avoid urolithiasis problems. Coccidiosis control may be necessary.

Day 20:

Provide clean water.

Day 25:

Reduce number of feeds to 2 on restricted feeding system.

Day 30:

Wean if on restricted feeding, restrict feeding if on ad libitum milk system. It is essential that solid food is kept clean by preventing lambs walking and defaecating in feed troughs.

Day 42:

Wean ad libitum fed group.

Day 80:

Ewe lambs for breeding can be turned out to grass, preferably 'clean', and fed restricted amounts of concentrates; at first 400g/day should be allowed but this should then be decreased to 200g/day after a few weeks.

Day 100 – 120:

Lambs will be ready for slaughter at 35-40kg, having grown at 300–400g/day from weaning and having consumed 85 – 100kg complete diet.

Lambs may also be removed from their dams at any time after they have reached 5 weeks of age and fed the complete diet. Performance figures should be similar to those stated above.

THIN EWES

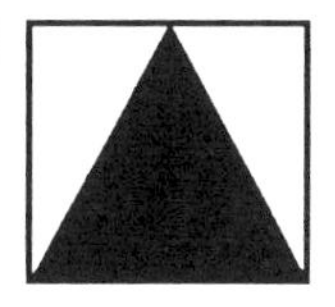

Thin ewes are interesting and important for the following reasons:

(1) They are common which should encourage us to do something about them.

(2) The causes are not infinite; in fact, for most cases, the list is short:

lack of food

inadequate teeth - particularly the cheek teeth

chronic lameness (joints rather than feet), *chronic* fascioliasis, *chronic* pneumonias

This should encourage us to diagnose them accurately.

(3) If there are many thin ewes, look first at the food and the number of foetuses or lambs; if there are a few, also look at the 'fangs' (teeth) and the faeces; if there are only one or two, also look at the limbs and the lungs.

(4) Thin ewes have suffered an insult for some time, which may imply irreversibility, i.e. they may not get better.

(5) Thin ewes aren't 'worth' much, but deserve a lot because they represent a serious welfare problem.

(6) Thin ewes are generally unprofitable, for the following reasons:

(a) if at tupping, they produce fewer lambs

(b) if in late pregnancy, they produce smaller lambs and risk pregnancy toxaemia

(c) if at lambing, they produce less colostrum and show less interest in their lambs, which in turn are more susceptible to disease.

(d) if in early lactation, they produce less milk leading to poor growth rate in their lambs.

CONDITION SCORING (CS)

One of the reasons for thin ewes being common is because the fleece masks their condition and it is only when the ewe is shorn or handled that the thinness is disclosed. Condition scoring was introduced to overcome this problem and is now an essential tool in good flock management as well as in the clinical examination of individual sick sheep.

The crucial element in the technique is to decide by feeling the mid-lumbar region, whether the ewe is "too thin" or "too thick" i.e. is it too bony or too fat, or just about right, so that action follows, for example, by separating and supplying extra, or sometimes, less food.

A number score (1–5) is given and is rather like marking exam papers. Score 3 is mid-way (50%) and is the pass mark but with nothing to spare. Score 1 fails badly because it is much too thin and score 5 is excessive! There are always disputes between markers, but they shouldn't differ by more than half a score. It needs practice across the full range of scores and standardising with other scorers from time to time, and each time it usually requires doing a few 'to get your hand in', but it is a technique that is learnt quickly and needs no kit, only one sensitive hand! There is a useful Trainee Guide published by the Agricultural Training Board, Beckenham BR3 4PB, and another good leaflet produced by the Meat and Livestock Commission, Milton Keynes, MK2 2EF.

Two vital times to condition score a flock are 6 to 8 weeks pre-tupping and 6 to 8 weeks pre-lambing, because then there is time to alter events by, for instance, re-allocating resources such as food, housing and shepherding. Repeat scoring in about 4 weeks is advisable because at least it will suggest what the future holds, although it may be too late by then to alter some of the events. Ewes with condition score of less than 3 should be separated and clinically checked. Most will require more and perhaps better food, whilst some will require treatment or even culling.

TEETH

It is very important to be able to examine sheep teeth properly not only for aging but also because faulty teeth are one of the most common causes for adult sheep to be thin.

Aging – a rough and ready guide

Age (years)	Incisors	Cheek teeth (one side)
Up to one (lamb, hog, wether)	4 pairs (8) temporary	3 premolars – temporary 2 molars – permanent
One to two (shearling/yearling)	1 pair permanent *(2 tooth)* 3 pairs temporary	3 premolars – permanent 3 molars – permanent
Two to three	2 pairs permanent *(4 tooth)* 2 pairs temporary	" "
Three to four	3 pairs permanent *(6 tooth)* 1 pair temporary	" "
Rising four and over (sometimes to a grand old age)	4 pairs permanent *(8 tooth = Full Mouth)*	" "
Old sheep (but see note 4)	Less than 4 pairs permanent *(Broken Mouth)*	

Note:

There is a lot of variation within and between flocks, and some confusing features:

(1) 8 worn permanent incisors can look like 8 temporaries and vice versa. Generally, the temporaries are smaller, more triangular and without a table.

(2) The permanent corner incisor is usually less obvious than the other permanent incisors (it sometimes never erupts). It can look like a temporary tooth, making the sheep appear like a 3-year-old (6 tooth).

(3) Age the sheep in relation to the time of year, e.g. in the autumn most sheep will be X years plus or minus 6 months, whilst in the spring they will be just X years.

(4) Periodontal disease causes premature incisor and molar tooth loss and sheep then look older than they really are.

(5) The 1st and 2nd molar (4th and 5th cheek teeth) are present early in the lambs' life and a year or more before the temporary premolars are shed and the permanent premolars erupt. The region between the 3rd premolar and the 1st molar is, therefore, a very susceptible site for food impaction and progressive disease, starting in the first year or so of life. It is almost certainly the reason why the mid-ramus is the area most prominently affected (lump and sinus) in periodontal disease of the cheek teeth.

Teeth Problems

Incisors

Very occasionally faulty eruption occurs and a Dentigerous Cyst may result which ultimately causes considerable bony deformity and the need for premature culling. Mal-position in relation to the dental pad (over or undershot) is quite common but it is probably not significant unless extreme. It has low hereditability, and the selection for good apposition (bite or occlusion) is unreliable before 3 years' old. Premature loss of incisors (Broken Mouth) is extremely common and is connected with PERIODONTAL DISEASE.

To some extent, tooth eruption always causes a local 'itis', but in many sheep, there is a serious progressive gingivitis leading to gum recession early in life, and subsequent loosening of teeth following subgingival plaque formation and periodontitis. Osteomyelitis, abscessation and sinus formation are natural consequences of the initial gum pathology. The reason for such serious progression is uncertain; the role of some oral bacteria, such as *Bacteroides gingivalis*, is under investigation and there is a strong suspicion that gritty food may be involved, which may help to explain why the prevalence of the disease is much higher on some farms than others, where the soil types and grazing environments differ. Sometimes, there is a family or breed prevalence within a flock, suggesting a genetic component.

Premature loss of incisors in hill and upland sheep probably reduces the ability of ewes to maintain body condition and to feed their lambs well, and so often results in premature culling. Its effect on lowland sheep is not so serious providing the cheek teeth are not involved, and therein lies the problem. Broken-mouthed sheep should always have their cheek teeth checked, because incisor loss often means molar loss, although occasionally, the incisors may appear healthy whilst the cheek teeth are not, so the customary reliance on incisor examination alone (aging) can be very misleading; the rule is that all thin sheep need their cheek teeth examining.

Cheek teeth

Make sure the ewe is facing the light (and have a good torch), and also have a good gag, e.g. block of bevelled hard wood 12 x 2 x 2cm (Shaw gag) or a metal sheep gag (Alfred Cox).

Before you look inside:

(1) Note CS, dribbling, staining of lips and mouth, mouthing (when trying to eat), quidding, swelling of cheeks with wads of food, and spilt quids and cuds on the ground.

(2) Feel along the outside of the cheek for evidence of pain (flinching on pressure), and for irregularity of teeth (shear mouth and wave mouth).

(3) Feel with finger and thumb along the two rami for bony swellings

(4) Note maxillary and mandibular sinuses.

(5) Note abdominal distension for ruminal 'impaction' and/or pregnancy (likely to develop pregnancy toxaemia).

Now look inside, and with the gag in place, note any gaps (particularly common in the lower jaw), irregularities, loose teeth, food impaction and spikes. Look particularly in the mid-third region (check teeth 3 and 4); If there are gaps, the corresponding upper (or lower) tooth lengthens through lack of wear, making it even more difficult and painful for the sheep to chew properly.

Treatment

(1) Assess whether it is worth doing anything other than cull. Some action usually must be taken on grounds of welfare as well as economics, but dentistry often provides only temporary relief and may only be indicated in pregnancy or near marketing.

(2) Remove obvious loose teeth under light anaesthesia (e.g. Sagatal, RMB Animal Health Ltd., approx. 1ml/5kg.) and inject long-acting antibiotic (e.g. Terramycin LA, Pfizer Ltd., 1ml/10kg) twice at 4 day interval. Ewes can thrive, given a chance, without any incisors ('gummers'), providing their cheek teeth are healthy. Molar rasping may have short-term advantage.

(3) Feed comfortable high quality concentrates and roughage, and separate from greedy competitors. Proprietary nuts are usually too hard. A useful mix is 40% whole barley, 40% sugar beet pulp, 17% soya and 3% minerals.

Control

(1) Check feeding and breeding. Fault in Ca/P, Vitamin D, Copper and Fluorine levels in the feed should be considered, as well as generally inadequate feeding which may lead to excessive soil eating (which compounds the problems of mineral deficiencies and gum irritation). The prevalence in a flock may suggest genetic factors, in which case the ram(s) or even the breed needs changing. Feeding blocks and roots may not promote incisor loss, but certainly require healthy teeth.

(2) 'Bite correction', sometimes called 'teeth grinding': This was introduced to conserve overgrown incisors for an extra 1 or 2 years. Full-mouthed ewes (3 to 4 years) with incisors overshooting the dental pad, are selected for correction. The tips of the incisors are ground and re-shaped just enough to allow them to meet snugly on the dental pad, using a battery-operated, high-speed grinder and special gag (Alfred Cox). The technique is quick (30–50 ewes/hour), and appears painless but the efficacy and welfare require long term evaluation. It has been declared illegal (1986) until this evaluation has been completed.

Further reading

Spence, A J (1987). 'The sheep's dental anatomy and broken mouth'. *Proceedings of the Sheep Veterinary Society* vol. 12, 1–8.

FASCIOLIASIS

Fascioliasis is of immense economic importance in sheep throughout the wetter western parts of Britain. No effective immunity develops and thus disease can occur in any age of sheep. A high proportion of the flock is usually affected.

Acute disease, associated with migrating immature flukes, is most commonly seen from October to February after a wet summer, and chronic fascioliasis, in which adults are found in the bile ducts, is seen from December to April. A sub-acute form of the disease has been described as occurring in December and January when a mixture of adult and immature flukes will be present. The best way to decide if a farm has liver fluke is to take faeces from 10-20 untreated thin ewes in December to May and look for eggs, though eggs are likely to be present all the year round in untreated ewes.

Acute fascioliasis

Sudden death may occur in epidemic years and the mortality can be very high. Affected animals may be seen with extreme weakness, severe anaemia (PCV 10%), abdominal pain and ascites. The liver is enlarged with haemorrhagic tracts. Eggs are not found in the faeces and there are usually over 1000 immature (0.5cm long) flukes in the substance of the liver. Acute disease is seen about 6 weeks after the ingestion of a large number of metacercariae.

The flock should be treated (see page 86) and moved to a clean pasture, wherever possible. The metacercariae will remain viable for several months, especially over the winter, so do not return sheep to the pasture containing an extensive snail habitat before the end of May.

Chronic fascioliasis

Affected animals show a progressive loss in condition proceeding to emaciation, and signs of anaemia will be present, since the PCV is usually about 15%. Mucous membranes are pale and the nictitating membrane is pale and oedematous (flukey-eye). Ascites often occurs but sub-mandibulary oedema ('bottle-jaw'), often described as being typical of chronic fascioliasis, is rare and does occur in other clinical conditions. Wool yield is reduced even in light infections, as is the milk production of ewes, thus resulting in reduced weight gain in the lambs. The liver is small and cirrhotic, the bile ducts enlarged and thickened. There are usually about 250 adult flukes present and eggs can be found in the faeces. The prepatent period is about 10 weeks.

Affected animals can be treated with a wide range of drugs (see page 86).

Prevention

This is based upon a knowledge of the environmental conditions which are needed to allow the development of the fluke from egg to infective metacercaria, on the ground and in the snail, *Lymnea truncatula*. This mud snail measures up to 7mm in length and the operculum is on the right side when held upright.

The most important cycle of infection involves the 'Summer' infection of snails which results in the main pasture infection with metacercariae occurring in September and October. The 'Winter' infection of snails occurs when snails become infected in October of one year and the life cycle is complete in May and June of the next year. This can give rise to acute fascioliasis in July and August rather than in the autumn. It is a rare occurrence in Britain because May is usually a dry month and the over-wintered snails commence to die off at this time.

Short-term control

The MAFF produces a liver fluke forecast in early autumn which should be used to avoid acute fascioliasis in epidemic years by preventing sheep ingesting large numbers of cercariae from September onwards by:

(1) Removal of sheep to a pasture with no snail habitats.

(2) Fencing off small habitats.

(3) Sheep should be kept away from habitats until May of the following year since metacercariae are long-lived during winter months. If sheep must be grazed on habitats during the winter in epidemic years, anthelmintics which are effective against very young flukes given at 4–6 week intervals may help in preventing serious disease.

Long-term control

This is based on:

(1) Improved drainage to eliminate snail habitats. ADAS drainage officers will survey and produce plans and grants are available for drainage in some areas.

(2) Prophylactic use of anthelmintics to reduce pasture contamination with eggs so that the proportion of infected snails is reduced.

(3) The use of molluscicides to limit snail populations, in May/June and/or August, is often recommended but, unfortunately, the most effective molluscicide, n-trityl-morpholine, is no longer available.

On many farms where habitats are few and small, eradication is possible by a logical combination of these principles.

A survey of snail habitats is essential before any of these control schemes can be developed; this may be done by ADAS drainage officers or by the private veterinary surgeon with a 6" map of the fields and an experienced eye for suitable snail habitats. Improvement of hill grazings with basic slag and lime increases the pH and allows previously unsuitable land to become very suitable for snail multiplication. Severe outbreaks of fascioliasis have been seen on these improved pastures where previously the acid pH of the peat prevented extensive habitats and the possible dangers of improvement of peaty pastures should be borne in mind.

Use of anthelmintics *(see page 86)*

Modern anthelmintics act against immature stages as well as against adults. Some drugs, such as diamphenethide and triclabendazole are effective against very early stages (1 or 2 weeks old), others against somewhat older, immature flukes (rafoxanide, brotianide and nitroxynil-4 to 6 weeks old) whilst some drugs are only effective against adults (oxyclozanide, albendazole). Closantel, whilst not being effective against very young flukes, prevents egg-laying by adult flukes for over 10 weeks. Diamphenethide and triclabendazole are obviously the drugs of choice in the treatment of acute fascioliasis. Drugs are also a very important part of any control programme, the aim of which is to prevent fluke eggs being passed by the sheep (or cattle) so that the infection rate of snails is greatly reduced. Field trials with rafoxanide have shown that if all adult sheep are treated in mid-April, followed by a second treatment six weeks later, the summer infection is reduced to a very low level. Further treatment in October and January reduced fluke burdens over a 3 year period to about 10% of pre-trial numbers, and resulted in considerable increase in wool yield and lamb productivity (The extra revenue from fleece sales was sufficient to pay for the anthelmintic treatments). This work was done in an area where fluke was widespread and habitats extensive, and in areas of lighter infection, it would probably be sufficient to treat in April, October and January. The advent of triclabendazole and closantel should allow similar results to be obtained with dosing at less frequent interval (10 weeks).

JOHNE'S DISEASE

This is an uncommon disease in sheep. It needs to be on one's list of causes of thinness in old ewes, although food, teeth, fascioliasis, chronic pneumonias and lameness are much more likely causes. However, it can become established in a closed flock, and a 10% incidence has been recorded in some flocks with an even higher prevalence in some abattoir surveys.

Diagnosis

The disease is similar to that in cattle but with the following variations:

(1) Scouring may not be so obvious, and may be intermittent with only soft faeces.

(2) As with most debilitating diseases of sheep, the fleece pulls out easily (wool break).

(3) As well as the bovine strain of *Mycobacterium johnei*, there is also the yellow pigmented strain which can be seen at PME, staining the intestine.

(4) The organisms are often not easily found in the faeces, and a necropsy and gut histology is required to establish the diagnosis.

(5) Individual complement-fixation tests are unreliable and really only for use as a flock test.

The typical story is of a few old, dirty-tailed and broken-woolled ewes which are unaccountably thin (feed and teeth OK), deteriorating soon after lambing.

Control

(1) Cull clinical cases and fatten their lambs for slaughter rather than keep for breeding.

(2) Vaccinate healthy lambs kept for breeding with 0.75ml of Ministry cattle vaccine.

(3) Ensure good control of other debilitating conditions, eg. lack of food, worms, fluke and cobalt which appear to predispose to the development of the clinical disease.

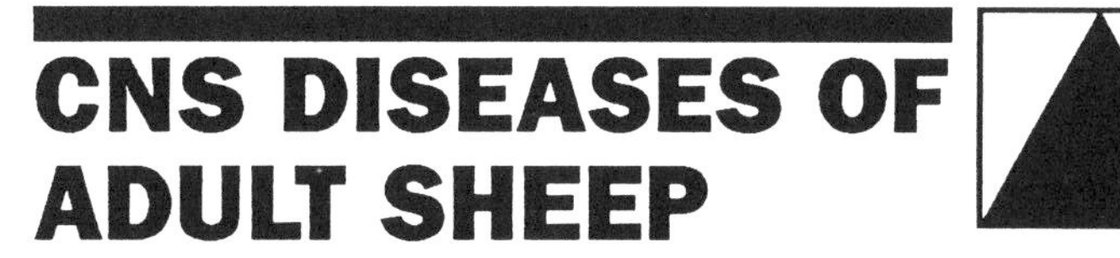

CNS DISEASES OF ADULT SHEEP

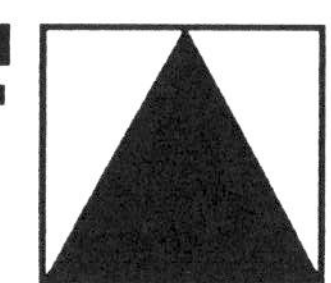

A CLINICAL APPROACH TO THE 3 'METABOLIC DISEASES' OF EWES (PREGNANCY TOXAEMIA, HYPOCALCAEMIA, HYPOMAGNESAEMIA)

These are a notoriously difficult group of conditions to cope with, mainly because they are difficult to differentiate clinically and they may co-exist, the farmer has often 'got there' first and confused the picture with various treatments as well as causing delay, a number of cases may occur at the same time, the results of treatment are often disappointing and prevention is not simple.However, if one tries to keep one's feet on the ground, some sort of logic can prevail which should lead to more satisfaction for the three parties.

Clinical Diagnosis (from USUAL findings)

Pregnancy Toxaemia (PT, Twin-lamb disease)

(1) Last month of pregnancy and before spring grass.

(2) Thin (C.S.2), much less commonly in overfat ewe.

(3) Insufficient food, which usually means concentrates. Usually for some weeks but may be sudden, e.g. following bad weather or movement.

(4) Old or appear old, due to broken mouth and molar problems.

(5) Large abdomen (2 or more lambs).

(6) Separated from the rest of the flock, easy to catch, blind and standing motionless, showing fine tremors leading to convulsions (on handling). Refuse feed.

(7) Urine (by smothering) – rapid and strong positive Ketotest suggests PT; negative makes it unlikely.

(8) If not treated, progressively worsens *over days* and dies.

Hypocalcaemia

(1) More common in late pregnancy rather than early lactation, in contrast to cattle.

(2) Often just been moved and not fed immediately before or after movement and therefore a number may be affected simultaneously.

(3) Typical signs of 'milk-fever' - ataxic, leading to recumbency, depression and atony (bloat, no faeces etc.) and loss of consciousness.

(4) If not treated, progressively worsens *over hours* and dies. Hypocalcaemia may be the precursor of PT.

Hypomagnesaemia

(1) Nearly always after lambing and either on lush grass (plenty of food) or bare pastures (insufficient food).

(2) Excitable, leading to convulsions and rapid death.

(3) Sometimes co-existing with hypocalcaemia (hence the confusion).

(4) If not treated, progressively worsens *over minutes* and dies.

Pre-treatment blood (where possible) can help retrospectively, but in practice, the diagnosis is more usually 'confirmed' by response (if any) to therapy.

Treatment

Needs to be prompt for all 3 conditions, otherwise the prognosis is hopeless; hence farmer therapy.

Pregnancy Toxaemia

(1) First day – 50–100ml glucose 40 i/v or s/c, and 150ml glucose electrolyte solution (e.g. Liquid Lectade, Beecham Animal Health) or 50ml propylene glycol (e.g. Ketol, Intervet UK Ltd) orally and repeat in a few hours. You hope that the ewe will begin to feed by then; if not, review your diagnosis and prognosis.

(2) Next day – if improving, continue with glucose until feeding well. If not improving, either slaughter or if less than 1 week before term, abort the lambs by 8ml (16mg) of beta or dexamethasone, or caesar (if lamb alive). Avoid repeated propylene glycol as it appears to lead to scouring.

Hypocalcaemia

20–40ml Ca20 i/v (where possible, but the lack of vascular tone does not make this easy!) and 50–100ml Ca20 s/c. You expect the ewe to respond like a cow with milk fever, eructating, defaecating and even 'walking off the needle'. If it does not respond, review your diagnosis.

Hypomagnesaemia

20ml CaMgP i/v (where possible) and 50ml $MgSO_4$ 25 s/c. N.B. NOT $MgSO_4$ 25 i/v. You hope that the ewe will quickly become less excitable and behave normally within an hour, but some equally quickly die.

If you are uncertain of the diagnosis at the first visit, a'rough and ready' approach is

(1) Pretreatment blood sample (green and grey tubes) for Ca/Mg/glucose/ketones estimations.

(2) i/v – 20–40ml CaMgP and 20–40ml glucose 20.

(3) s/c – 50–100ml CaMgP.

(4) Oral – 150 ml glucose electrolyte.

Control

Pregnancy Toxaemia

(1) Supply more concentrates to all sheep below C.S.3 (split and remove shy feeders) and reduce the hay.

(2) Green grass where possible.

(3) Shelter.

(4) In future, regularly C.S. in last 2 months of pregnancy, splitting off thin sheep for special attention. Select the best forage for late pregnancy.

(5) The season with the lush autumn (therefore, high ovulation rate) and hard winter is the one which can create the worst problems.

Hypocalcaemia

(1) Watch the flock after movement and have Ca injection handy.

(2) Provide hay and concentrates before leaving and on arrival.

(3) Increase the calcium and the Vit.D in the ration during the last 6 weeks of pregnancy.

Hypomagnesaemia

(1) Watch the flock after movement onto lush or bare fields and have $MgSO_4$ injection handy.

(2) If on lush pasture, move to poorer, until Mg supplement added.

(3) Feed extra magnesium (up to 14g Mg0 per day) via:

(a) Magnesium enriched cake or

(b) Magnesium enriched feed blocks or molasses licks (less reliable than (a)) or

(c) Magnesium bullets (Rumbul Sheep, Agrimin Ltd.), approx. £1.00 per ewe just before turnout.

(4) Give extra food to those which are under-fed.

(5) Shelter.

LISTERIOSIS

This is a sporadic disease of sheep (and less commonly, cattle) seen in one or other of the following forms:

(1) Encephalitis - by far the most common and significant form.

(2) Abortion.

(3) Diarrhoea and septicaemia.

(4) A few reports of kerato-conjunctivitis and also mastitis.

(5) Septicaemia and death in young lambs.

There has been an increase in reported incidents of listeriosis in the UK from 101 in 1980 to 434 in 1987, and it is now one of the most common causes of sporadic disease in individual adult sheep, particularly in the late winter months when silage is being fed and teeth are changing. It is assumed that silage feeding has much to do with this increased incidence, for it is well established that poor quality silage, particularly if it is contaminated with soil, and stored where air can get at it, can contain large doses of *Listeria monocytogenes*. It is thought that the organism gains entry via any mouth lesions, e.g. changing teeth, and travels up the V and/or VII cranial nerves to involve the meninges and mid-brain, or via the alimentary tract to involve the pregnant uterus in ewes and cause septicaemia in young lambs.

Clinical signs

The alimentary form often produces diarrhoea and even brief general illness, and if the ewe is pregnant, abortion may follow a week or so later, sometimes with retention of foetal membranes and subsequent systemic illness.

The much more common central nervous form appears to have a longer incubation period, cases usually occurring about six weeks after silage is fed. It is mainly a winter disease with a peak incidence in February/March, when many ewes are pregnant. The signs are variable but classically there is unilateral VII cranial nerve paralysis, which may show as a drooping ear, eyelid and lip with consequent dribbling and difficulty in eating and drinking. It also means that the animal is unable to respond to the menace test which may mislead one into thinking that the ewe is blind in that eye, and so confuse the condition with, for example, gid. If the face and lip and gum are tapped or pinched, there is often a loss of sensation on that side indicating paralysis of the cranial nerve. The ewe also often shows a head aversion and a one-side stiff neck and she circles in one direction and may fall over onto one side. Usually, the ewe is noticeably very disturbed, ranging from the depressed to the convulsive. Deterioration usually occurs over just a few days, leading to recumbency and death.

Diagnosis

(1) The CNS form requires differentiating clinically (if you can!) from such conditions as pregnancy toxaemia, gid, CCN and abscessation. Brain histology is necessary for confirmation. Serology is not helpful.

(2) The alimentary/abortion form requires faeces, vaginal discharges, foetuses and milk (if any) for culture and paired blood sample for serology.

(3) If, as expected, silage is being fed, or was fed some time during the last six weeks, examine it for 'rotten' material. Most silage contains some *Listeria*, although very rotten silage may be sterile.

(4) Be very careful when handling suspect material, including silage, particularly if you are pregnant or unwell.

Treatment

The organism is sensitive to a wide range of antibiotics but therapy is usually disappointing. Success is more likely if treatment is early and vigorous, which means high dose given i/v initially, and at least twice daily for up to 14 days! (e.g. Trivetrin Injection, 3ml/50kg, Coopers Pitman-Moore).

Anti-inflammatory treatment given i/v is also indicated such as flunixin (Finadyne Solution,1ml/50kg – Kirby-Warwick Animal Health) or dimethyl sulphoxide (DMSO, 50ml A.R. grade in 500ml glucose-saline/50kg), though the latter is not licensed for veterinary use. Anti-convulsants given i/v may also be required such as diazepam or phenobarbitone (Gardenal sodium, RMB), given to effect.The common unilateral eye complications of corneal ulceration and uveitis also require intensive local therapy, supported sometimes by suturing the lids.

Further reading
Milne, Elspeth M, (1989). 'Management of Bacterial Infections of the CNS of Sheep', *Proceedings of the Sheep Veterinary Society. Vol. 14 (in press).*

Control

(1) Silage:

Although a few incidents do occur at pasture, most follow silage feeding. It is almost impossible to avoid contamination by *Listeria*, so one must seek to avoid conditions in which it multiplies.

Suggestions:

(a) Make high quality silage with a pH<5 and a D value >65%, with additives where necessary. Avoid gross soil contamination, e.g. mole hills, by not cutting too short, so that it has an ash content of <100g/kg DM.

(b) Compact and completely seal the silage, and so avoid air getting into the sides and tops of clamps and through insecure polythene (including bales).

(c) Avoid feeding rotten silage, which can be seen and smelt on the top or sides, as a layer or even in lumps in the middle, or left over in the troughs.

(d) It is less risky to feed suspect silage to cattle.

(e) Consider injecting long-acting antibiotic, e.g. oxytetracycline, if the incidence is alarming.

(2) Aborting ewes:

As always, isolate and clean up after (be careful).

(3) Vaccination

Not yet available, but live attenuated vaccines are available on the continent and look promising if used selectively.

COENURIASIS (GID, STURDY, BENDRO)

This is one of the most common causes of disease of the central nervous system in sheep. The causative agent is the metacestode (larval) stage of the life-cycle of *Taenia multiceps, (Coenurus cerebralis)*, a tapeworm occurring in the dog.

The adult cestode also occurs in the fox but the worms seldom reach maturity and become gravid and foxes should not be blamed until every possible dog source of infection has been considered. The metacestode is also recorded in cattle, goats, horses, deer and man, but at a much lower incidence than in sheep.

The larvae migrate in the bloodstream throughout the body but can only continue their development within the CNS. Over a period of 2 to 8 months, the Coenurus grows into a fluid-filled cyst containing around one hundred scoleces. Multiple cysts rarely occur in natural infections, possibly because an established cyst inhibits the development of further cysts.

Dogs usually acquire the infection either through scavenging dead sheep, or through being fed sheep heads obtained from abattoirs. Surveys have shown that about 5 to 10% of farmdogs in the British Isles are affected with the adult tapeworm and that they carry a mean worm burden of about 10 adults.

Clinical signs

Acute coenuriasis usually goes unnoticed. Some 2–4 weeks after a sheep has ingested a large number of the tapeworm eggs, there is the development of nervous signs such as ataxia, blindness, muscle tremors, nystagmus, excitability and collapse. Diagnosis is extremely difficult and is usually at post mortem examination where haemorrhagic tracts and migrating parasites are found in the brain. The chronic form of the disease is much more frequently seen. The onset of clinical signs is usually 3 to 8 months after infection.The affected animal shows a variety of neurological deficits usually correlating closely with the location of the cyst within the CNS. About 80% of cysts are located in the cerebrum, 10% in the cerebellum, 5% are multiple cysts in several locations and the remainder are in the brainstem and spinal cord.

Affected sheep are usually identified initially by the farmer because of abnormal behaviour in the flock such as standing apart or failing to respond to the dog. Neurological examination should then reveal specific localising signs, although it is important to consider combinations of signs rather than relying too heavily on any one deficit and if a farmer has become very good at recognising early behavioural abnormalities, other neurological signs may not be very obvious.

Clinical sign	Interpretation
Behaviour:	
Depression	Rostral cerebrum.
Excitability	Temporal (lateral) cerebrum.
Posture and Movement:	
Circling – wide circle	Ipsilateral cerebrum.
– tight circles	Contralateral cerebrum (lateral ventricle or basal nuclei). Evidence of circling may be a plait of straw wound around hind leg on inside of circle. Some brainstem cysts may induce circling.
Postural deficits, e.g. wheelbarrow and hemiwalking tests	Contralateral cerebrum. Bilateral deficits may indicate cerebellum.
Dysmetria (usually hypermetria)	Cerebellum.

Vision and Eye Movement

Unilateral blindness	Contralateral caudal cerebrum (occipital lobe). There is an 89% crossover of optic axons in the sheep, so that some deficit (in the nasal visual field) may be found in the ipsilateral eye.
Bilateral blindness	Some cerebellar cysts block the menace reflex, either unilaterally or bilaterally.
Nystagmus	Cerebellum or vestibular nuclei. Brainstem cysts involving the vestibular pathways may induce a spontaneous nystagmus. Nystagmus of cerebellar origin is induced by eye movement.
Strabismus	Brainstem nuclei of cranial nerves III, IV and VI. The trochlear nerve (IV) crosses the midline so that the dorsomedial deviation of the eye is contralateral.

Head Position:

Head tilt – head rotated but nose points forwards	Vestibular or cerebellovestibular structures or pathways. The cyst is usually on the same side as the tilt, i.e. the side of the lower ear.
Head aversion – head rotated and nose averted to either side and usually downwards	Cerebrum. The direction of the head aversion is not a reliable guide to the location of the cyst.
Raised/lowered head	Dorsiflexion of the neck, especially in the recumbent animal (opisthotonus), can occur when the cyst is in the cerebellum. The head is often held downwards, and there is resistance to neck extension, when the cyst is in the rostral cerebrum.
Head tremor	An intention tremor may be seen during movement of the head when there is involvement of the cerebellum.

As the cyst develops, the clinical signs gradually increase in extent and severity, progressing to recumbency and death (over days or weeks) if the cyst is not removed surgically.

Differential diagnosis

Coenuriasis usually occurs sporadically, although occasionally outbreaks are seen. The disease is characterised by the slowly progressive development of CNS signs in sheep over 4 months old (usually 1 to 2 years and very rarely over 3).

Listeriosis is an acute disease (2 to 3 days), often with facial paralysis, occurring as mini-outbreaks mainly in winter, and usually associated with silage feeding.

CCN is also an acute disease (1 to 3 days), resulting in staggering gait, tremor and fits, but responding to early therapy with thiamine.

Louping-ill is a febrile illness characterised by 'leaping' movements and usually occurring as outbreaks amongst yearlings in tick areas and in tick season (Spring/Autumn).

Other conditions to be considered include CNS abscess, swayback, intracranial injury, Border Disease, scrapie, pregnancy toxaemia, hypocalcaemia and hypomagnesaemia.

A differential white cell count and an analysis of cerebrospinal fluid may aid diagnosis. Usually, the white cell picture is not altered by coenuriasis so that a neutrophilia or a crossover will generally indicate another cause of the CNS signs, e.g. listeriosis or abscess, but these changes do not occur invariably. CSF sampling should be carried out with care in cases where a raised intracranial pressure is suspected (e.g. coenuriasis); only 0.5 ml should be taken from the lumbar cistern to avoid herniation of the cerebellum. In coenuriasis, the CSF does not show any diagnostic changes; surprisingly, there is no eosinophilia.

The chronic nature of the disease and age of affected animals, together with a known farm incidence, will aid diagnosis. In addition, the presence of skull softening at or near the horn bud site, due to the intracranial pressure, is diagnostic but is not a reliable guide to the localisation of the cyst.

Treatment

Lambs near killing weight should be sent for slaughter. Surgical removal of the cyst should be attempted in breeding animals or those too small for slaughter. With practice, the surgical success rate is as high as 80%.

General anaesthesia is obtained with i/v pentobarbitone (Sagatal, RMB Animal Health Ltd.) at a dose of approximately 0.44 ml per kg body weight although it is worth remembering that in an animal with raised intracranial pressure, the dose will be reduced by about one-third of the calculated amount. Prior to surgery, crystalline penicillin (1.5g) and dexamethasone (6mg) should be given intravenously, although it is wise to omit the steroid when dealing with a pregnant ewe. A C-shaped skin incision is made just caudal to the horn bud on the appropriate side (L or R cerebral cortex), or in the mid line just rostral to the nuchal line (cerebellum) (Fig 1). The skull is trephined (0.5–1.5cm diameter) and a circular plate of bone removed (Fig 2). Sometimes, the skull is so soft that scissors may be used. However, it is not safe to assume that the site of skull softening indicates the location of the cyst. The bone at the cerebellar site is at least 0.5cm thick and may bleed. In trephining at the cerebellar site, it is important to avoid the transverse suture line about 1.5cm rostral to the nuchal line, since this marks the position of the tentorium cerebelli and the transverse sinus and serious haemorrhage could follow. The meninges are cut and reflected to expose the cerebrum, which will bulge due to increased intracranial pressure. A 16 gauge needle and cannula (e.g. horse i/v catheter) is inserted. When the cyst is punctured, clear cyst fluid wells up the needle. The needle is removed and a 20–50 ml syringe is attached to the cannula and most of the fluid is withdrawn. Cerebral cysts average 35ml but may contain over 100ml; cerebellar cysts contain 10–25ml. Suction is used to trap the pale grey cyst wall in the end of the cannula which is then elevated to allow the pedicle of cyst wall to be grasped with artery forceps. Gentle tension is then applied until the wall is removed, draining more fluid from the cyst if required. The depth of the trephine hole at the cerebellar site may reduce the angulation of the cannula, making it difficult to grasp a cyst that is laterally situated in the cerebellum. Only the skin incision is sutured, and antibiotic cover is continued for 2 more days. The sutures are removed in 10 days and the skull heals in about 1 month.

The results of surgery can be very rewarding, the animal returning to apparent normality within 7 days in the majority of cases.

Control

(1) Worm dogs with a drug which is effective against cestodes e.g. praziquantel (Droncit, Bayer UK Ltd.) at least as frequently as every 3 months.

(2) Do not feed uncooked sheep heads to dogs.

(3) Dispose of sheep carcases properly.

(4) Avoid sheep grazing heavily infected pasture e.g. following sheepdog trials or used by hounds.

Other tapeworms with larval stages in sheep

Dogs act as definitive hosts for several other tapeworms whose metacestode stage occurs in sheep. *Taenia hydatigena* is very common in sheepdogs and the larval stage, *Cysticercus tenuicollis,* occurs on the serosal surface of the liver and in the omentum in about 50% of lambs. Heavy infections are seen occasionally causing sudden death in young, usually pet, lambs. The liver is full of haemorrhagic tracts. Cysts cause some local condemnation of livers.

T.ovis has a larval stage in sheep muscles and heavy infection may result in carcase condemnation.

Echinococcus granulosus, a minute adult worm, gives rise to large hydatid cysts in livers and lungs, resulting in condemnation of offal. Clinical signs are not seen in sheep but hydatid disease is an important zoonosis in sheep rearing areas in central Wales.

Regular treatment of sheepdogs should be a component of sheep health programmes.

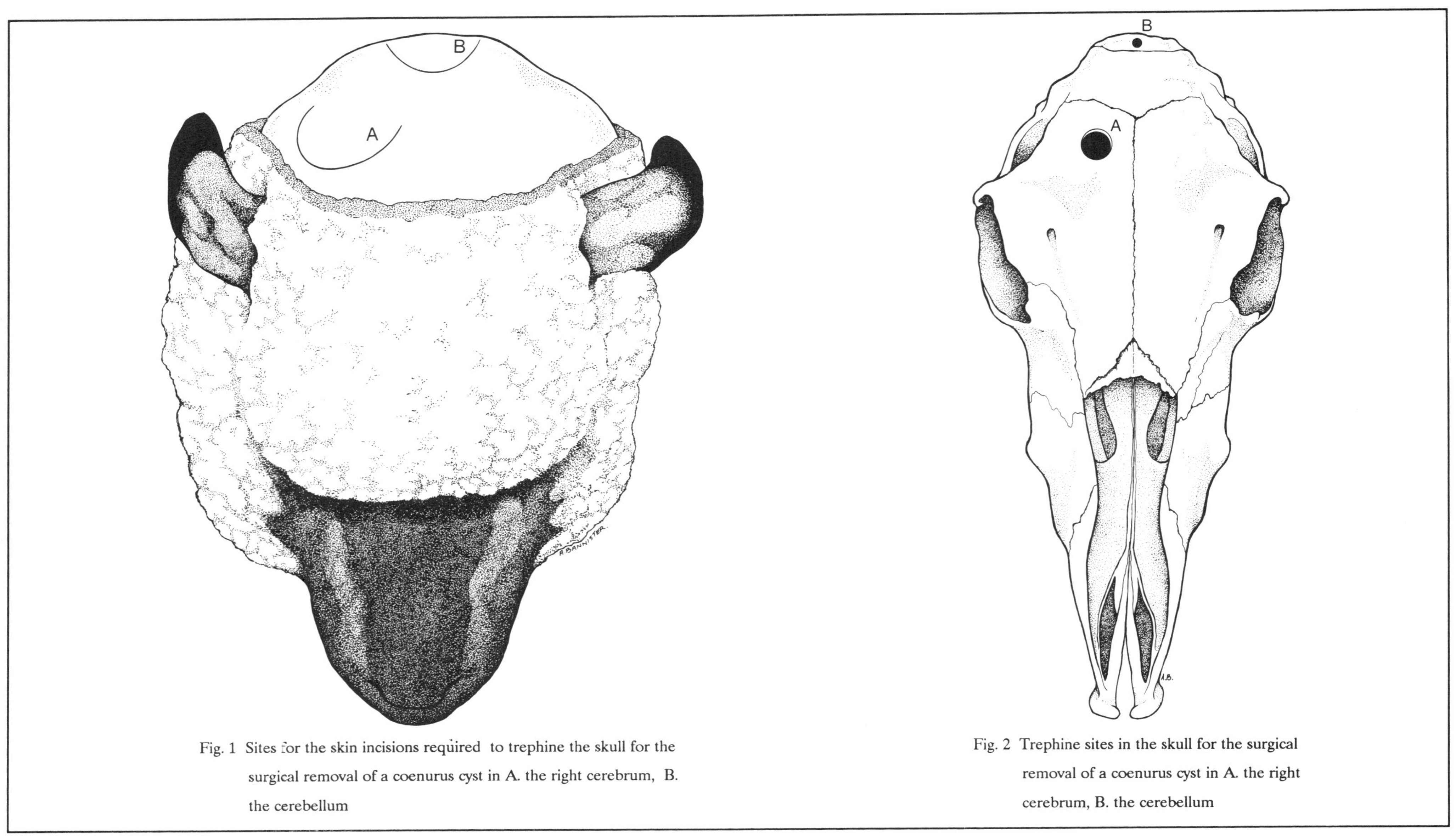

Fig. 1 Sites for the skin incisions required to trephine the skull for the surgical removal of a coenurus cyst in A. the right cerebrum, B. the cerebellum

Fig. 2 Trephine sites in the skull for the surgical removal of a coenurus cyst in A. the right cerebrum, B. the cerebellum

SCRAPIE

This chronic progressive degenerative central nervous disease of adult sheep (and goats) appears to be widespread, as individual cases keep 'popping up' in flocks throughout the country. Usually just one or two cases occur from year to year in a flock and so the disease is of little commercial importance to the average commercial sheep farmer producing prime lambs, but for the pedigree breeder where older sheep may be retained and where there is a susceptible strain, the incidence may be significant and a conspiracy of silence often exists, with the breeder culling cases on suspicion and the true incidence never revealed. Young breeding sheep are then sold which, unknown to the breeder and purchaser, are incubating the disease, which do not show clinically for months or years.

The causal agent has not been isolated, but it is very resistant to heat, formalin and UV light, which has serious implications for the control of the disease, including sterilisation of meat and offal. It is probably transmitted prenatally as well as laterally in the lambing pens and fields, and some breed lines appear to have a genetic susceptibility, hence the culling of particular families and rams. This genetic susceptibility seems to determine the Scrapie incubation period (Sip gene), so that, for example, homozygous recessive sheep (sip/sip) have a much prolonged incubation period, even beyond the natural life span of the sheep, whilst those with the dominant Sip gene show signs some years earlier.

Clinical signs

Clinical signs probably depend on which strain of the agent is involved and one strain may dominate in a flock and then only one clinical picture is evident.

(1) The most common and obvious sign is scratching, rubbing, sucking and nibbling fleece in an adult sheep (usually over 3 years). It is often seen at first as restlessness with the sheep darting about from place to place (trough to trough) as if it has been bitten, and turning to nibble anywhere it can get at, as well as rubbing on posts and walls etc (watching a case one could imagine it feels like 'prickly heat'). If one rubs the sheep, it responds by standing still and nibbling its lips in apparent pleasure and relief. (Note that this test is applicable for all conditions causing pruritis and is not diagnostic of scrapie).

    The rubbing leads to a loss of fleece or hair over any area which the sheep can get at, including the head and both sides of flank and hindlegs. A fine rough stubble is left, often with scabs.

(2) Some show an obvious change in temperament but without obvious skin irritation, the sheep appearing wild and excitable, and with it an incoordination, so that the sheep becomes awkward to catch and to examine, and it won't relax and allow its head to be held comfortably, and swallowing is sometimes difficult. Rams can be quite dangerous and the difficulty in raising the head can suggest a high cervical lesion e.g. from fighting. Some other cases just look dazed and depressed and don't appear to focus properly.

(3) Over the weeks and sometimes months, all these signs worsen although there is sometimes a temporary stasis or even remission; all become progressively thinner and die. Some appear to worsen after resting e.g. overnight, but after being helped up they become more mobile and alert.

Treatment

The condition is always fatal, so one should cull as soon as possible. The carcase should be buried or burnt to avoid getting into any food chain, but there is no legislation yet to enforce this. PME at VI centre is one way out of this difficulty.

Diagnosis

The clinical signs are eventually diagnostic but one obviously has to rule out primary skin conditions (e.g. sheep scab!) and all the other disorders affecting adult sheep! Brain histology is required for confirmation; there are no serological tests.

Control

(1) Slaughter and effectively dispose of the affected animal, preferably before lambing.

(2) Do not breed from any offspring.

(3) Look at the family line including the ram and remove it, but only where the problem is sufficiently important.

(4) Lamb any suspects in isolation and burn or bury foetal membranes.

(5) Join the MAFF Sheep and Goat Health Scheme which monitors disease via clinical cases and cull ewes.

The whole situation regarding scrapie has become much more complicated and high profile with the advent of a similar disease in cattle (Bovine Spongiform Encephalopathy-BSE). There is strong suspicion that material, brains in particular, from scrapie-infected sheep carcases, was responsible via concentrate food for this disease and a not unreasonable view is now expressed that such material has also been fed back to sheep and accounts for the apparent increase in incidence of scrapie and the suspicion that the disease is appearing in younger adult sheep; it is even suggested that scrapie should be renamed Ovine Spongiform Encephalopathy (OSE).

A further complication is the uncertainty about the possibility of the agent causing disease in humans and other animals, again via contaminated food. The current legislation concerning the control of BSE reflects, to some extent, these concerns.

Further reading

Barlow, R (1983). 'Neurological disorders of cattle and sheep', *In Practice*, Vol. 5, 77–84.
Barlow, R (1987). 'Differential diagnosis of nervous diseases of sheep', *In Practice*, Vol. 9, 76–81.

LAMENESS

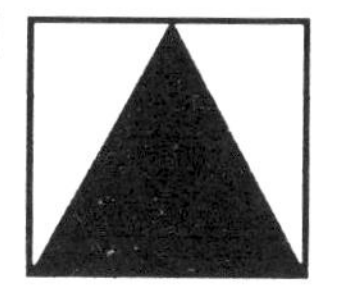

Lameness is so common in most flocks of sheep that many farmers regard it as a 'fact of life' and give it only irregular attention. Apart from the discomfort to the sheep, the loss in production can be considerable, eg. 0.5 kg/week in the fattening lamb, and inadequate food intake by the pregnant and lactating ewes, contributing to pregnancy toxaemia and neo-natal diseases.

Foot rot in all its forms is generally the most important condition causing lameness in sheep, but examination of a number of lame sheep in a flock will usually reveal a number of other causes, e.g.

(1) Interdigital problems caused by soil and grass 'balling', and by hyperplasia.

(2) Necrotic tracks and pus in the foot wall (as in cattle and pigs).

(3) Gross overgrowth leading to splitting and exposure of sensitive structures.

Although, again as in pigs and cattle, the foot is the most common site for cause of lameness, there are a number of important conditions affecting other parts of the limbs, e.g.

(1) Injury-various.

(2) Joint ill-various ages and causes.

(3) Post-dipping.

(4) Orf – Strawberry foot rot (see page 101/102).

(5) Muscular dystrophy (see page 43).

The prevalence of lameness in a flock varies greatly with climate, pasture, age and intensification e.g. over 50% of lowland lambs can be lame with foot rot if the weather and pasture conditions are suitable, whereas the prevalence in hill flocks is nearly always low; similarly, many lowland sheep may be lame with soil balling, a condition which rarely occurs in hill sheep.

FOOT CONDITIONS

Foot Rot

This is an infectious disease of the foot, starting as a superficial interdigital dermatitis with subsequent separation of the horn. It causes much lameness and merits more vigorous attention than it often gets. Whilst it does not cause such severe lameness as those conditions which involve joints, and on its own does not lead to thin sheep, foot rot can reduce food intake and cause some loss of condition and thus threaten production. It is obviously very painful and is of great significance from a welfare viewpoint.

Cause

The synergistic activity of *Bacteroides nodosus* and *Fusobacterium necrophorum* invading softened or injured interdigital skin and further aggravated by secondary organisms such as spirochaetes and corynebacteria. There are many strains of *B. nodosus* and they vary in their invasiveness.

Some clinically important features of the 'Fusiformis' bacteria

F. necrophorum: Environmental organism with many hosts, and therefore an ever-present risk.

B. nodosus: Confined to the feet and, for short periods (up to 2 weeks), on the ground. Eradication can be contemplated.

Both require warmth and moisture (seasonal incidence).

Both are anaerobic (exposed by paring and try not to bandage).

Both are sensitive to chemicals (easily killed).

Both cause a smelly, superficial necrosis (diagnostic lesions).

They complement each other (useful to control only one).

Clinical Picture

Often at least two feet (rarely all four: cf. F & M) are involved at the same time, leading, for example, to walking on both knees ('praying') with consequent rubbing and loss of hair over carpuses. Sheep with foot rot can run about and are not easy to catch in a field, and it is often difficult to pick out individually affected sheep, when a group are penned together, without turning all the sheep up and that is very tiresome and time-consuming.

All types start in the interdigital skin, and show as a moist hairless raw area extending to both digits. The condition at this stage is similar to foul in the foot of cattle but without the obvious soft tissue swelling and degree of pain and is identical to Scald.

Feet that are infected with the less invasive strains of *B. nodosus* show separation of the soft horn at the heel, whilst the most virulent strains invade across the sole, separating insensitive from sensitive horn and, if left unchecked, separation will continue up the walls to the coronary band, with consequent shedding of portions of the horn. This active separation, or under-running rather than destruction of tissues, facilitates paring, and as deep sensitive structures are rarely involved and secretory tissues are not irreversibly damaged, self-cure does occur. There is, however, little naturally induced immunity and, therefore, re-infection is common, and feet may show more than one stage of the disease.

There is usually a soft, sometimes black, cheese-like accumulation of debris between the layers, with the supposedly characteristic smell of necrosis found in foot rot.

The under-running that results from foot rot infection needs to be distinguished from the very common simple overgrowth of the outer wall and toe, where no sensitive tissues are involved and the sheep are not lame. Such overgrown horn provides a flap under which soil etc. gets impacted and it is argued that this predisposes to foot rot and/or white line disease. Unfortunately, routine flock foot-paring is usually directed at this overgrowth and foot rot cases are not selected out either then or between times for the delicate paring which they require.

A condition affecting only the interdigital skin is called Ovine Interdigital Dermatitis (OID) or SCALD. This probably results from infection by *F.necrophorum* without the synergistic presence of *B.nodosus*. The lesion appears the same as the primary stage of foot rot but little horny separation follows. It sometimes occurs as outbreaks in young lambs grazing on wet or icy pasture, causing substantial lameness; it can also be a considerable problem in housed sheep if the straw yards are wet and warm. It rapidly responds to spraying or foot bathing, but is not controlled by the current foot rot vaccines.

Clinically, this all adds up to the following:

(1) If there is considerable horn involvement, then severe foot rot is present and paring is important, as well as other treatments.

(2) If the separation is confined to the heels in all cases, then a less invasive form of *B. nodosus* is present, and foot bathing will be more essential than foot paring.

(3) If the lesions are confined to the interdigital structures then Scald is present; spraying and foot bathing will be useful but more reliance will be placed on dry weather/bedding.

(4) If a mixture of lesions are discovered (this is the most common finding) then a mixture of strains and organisms is probably present and a mixture of treatment is necessary, and vaccination should be considered.

Prevalence

This varies with rainfall and temperature, and also the concentration of sheep's feet. It is highest in warm wet weather when there are many ewes and lambs together, i.e. lowland flocks in spring and autumn, and it can be artificially induced by wet bedding indoors (housed sheep). It is probably lowest in hill sheep where concentration is least and temperatures low (plus the additional factor that the acid peat soil may not support Fusiforms).

Treatment

(1) Individual lame sheep

Careful paring of all under-run horn and spray with a tetracycline aerosol. Where possible, avoid bandaging and avoid causing haemorrhage. In particular, avoid excessive paring of the toe, which is a common site for an enlarging granuloma which causes severe lameness and requires excision and several dressings.

(2) The flock

Walk very slowly (several minutes) through a well-designed long, narrow foot-bath, after careful paring of all under-run feet, and keep in a concrete drying pen for 15 minutes. Use 10% zinc sulphate (Golden Hoof– Sheep Fair Products), and repeat weekly as required. Formalin is cheaper but more toxic to both the shepherd and the sheep and very painful to sheep with severe foot lesions. Zinc sulphate will penetrate the horn if the feet are soaked for some time (up to 1 hour) in a large footbath. The penetration is increased with the addition of a detergent (Footrite – C-Vet Ltd). This procedure is expensive and time-consuming in large flocks, but there is evidence that even without paring, foot rot can be eliminated by its diligent use.

(3) Severe cases and valuable stock (e.g. rams, heavily pregnant ewes)

One large dose (20mg/kg) of penicillin and streptomycin i/m, e.g.10ml Streptopen – Coopers Pitman-Moore, plus paring and foot spray.

Control

1. Most shepherds routinely trim and foot bath, but there is often no planned control and sheep and the shepherd learn to live with foot rot.The more energetic the programme, the more effective is the control.

2. Vaccination

There are two vaccines available from Coopers Pitman-Moore – 'Clovax' – costing approx. 50p/dose, and 'Footvax' – costing approx £1/dose and containing more strains of *B. nodosus*; it also has an oily adjuvant which causes a noticeable lump that usually recedes over a few weeks, although some will abscessate. Both require 2 doses initially and must be boosted twice a year. It is wise to vaccinate ewes at the beginning of any lengthy housing period, and early in pregnancy rather than late because this avoids wasting antibody in the colostrum to relatively unsusceptible young lambs.

Where the incidence of foot rot is high, vaccination should be seriously considered both for the sake of the sheep and the pocket. The exact schedule needs working out for each farm, and needs to be used in conjunction with foot paring and foot-bathing; it is not a substitute for these tried and trusted methods. New recombinant vaccines are being tested which should avoid the severe tissue reactions and perhaps induce a stronger immunity.

Eradication

Foot rot has been eradicated in some flocks but it is a difficult and time-consuming exercise and by no means certain. It certainly requires that the farmer be prepared to examine all feet, effectively pare and foot-bath, repeating the procedures at least once, and isolate or even cull persistent cases. Eradication implies safeguards against re-introduction and this means self-contained flocks (including adequate sheep fencing) or inspection and eradication of infection in purchased sheep. Few flocks, particularly the large ones, can manage all this. It is best to attempt it when most of the lambs have been marketed and old ewes culled, but before tupping. It is also wise to choose a time when there are few cases, brought about perhaps by a previous vaccination programme.

Further reading
Morgan, K (1987). 'Footrot', *In Practice*, Vol. 9, 124–29.

Foot Abscess

A variety of lesions occur which affect the wall of the foot, similar to those found in pigs and cattle. The lesions are usually a local necrotic laminitis with secondary abscessation and eventual bursting at the coronary band. Usually only one digit is involved, which is very painful when squeezed. Treat initially by paring and intensive systemic antibiotic therapy, i.e. high dose, twice daily for 1 week. Very severe and valuable cases, e.g. rams and pedigree stock, may justify irrigating the joint via a cannula inserted, for example, interdigitally through to a lateral coronary band sinus. X-rays help to decide if the joint (P.2/P.3) is involved, as does a probe and the degree of swelling and lameness (usually 10/10). Amputation, which is relatively cheap and easy, should also be considered.

Interdigital 'Fibromas'

Proud, fibrous outgrowths in the interdigital space (mainly hind feet) are a feature of some breeds e.g. Suffolk rams are notorious. Lameness occurs only when they become ulcerated and infected. Frequent foot-bathing maintains some control, but the worst cases require simple surgical removal under local anaesthesia; this is not a job to be done just before tupping!

Red Foot Disease of Lambs

This is an unusual condition of complete shedding of the horn from one or more digits in very young lambs and often complicated by corneal and mouth ulcers and shedding of horn buds. The incidence is seldom higher than 1% and is thought to be genetic rather than infectious. It is a persistent feature in some pure-bred flocks. Lambs become severely lame from damage to sensitive structures and require euthanasia. The disease resembles similar genetic disturbances, e.g. Epitheliogenesis imperfecta, in other species such as cattle, foals and kittens, but is probably not identical.

JOINT INFECTIONS

Young lambs up to 1 month - mainly lowland

Following a septicaemia, commonly of *Streptococcus dysgalactiae* or *Escherichia coli* via navel, tonsils or gut, there is a polysynovitis and arthritis, particularly of the stifle (soft, bulging and painful synovia in the patella region), carpus and hock joints, causing a reluctance to move about, with flexed joints and arched back; the lambs appear crouched and crippled. It is best to assume an *E. coli* infection and treat accordingly and vigorously. Standard methods of control for *E.coli* are indicated, but it is not always easy, nor is it always obvious what is at fault. 'Coliovac' (Hoechst Animal Health), a polyvalent *E.coli* vaccine administered twice to pregnant ewes, is worth considering in future if the incidence justifies the expense and if a laboratory has confirmed the diagnosis.

Lambs over 2 months - lowland

Stiff lambs/Erysipelas arthritis

On some farms, a significant number of fattening lambs at grass show a stiff, stilted, short-striding walk or hopping run, appearing to be lame on more than one leg.Very careful examination and palpation discloses some synovial swelling and pain in some limb joints, particularly stifle, hock and carpus. The condition is insidious and often irreversible by the time it is recognised. *Erysipelothrix insidiosa (rhusiopathiae)* is the 'favourite' organism causing a chronic fibrinous synovitis and arthritis. Often the organism cannot be isolated from the joints but a blood titre of 1/320 and over indicates the infection. Penicillin, preferably containing a long-acting component, is probably the drug of choice and it is tempting to use corticosteroids. (Such lame sheep need housing so that more intensive treatment and feeding can be applied and where they do not have to walk far for food or shelter. Repeated penicillin treatment is advisable.) Vaccination (eg. Erysorb ST-Hoechst Animal Health), may be indicated, including vaccinating ewes in late pregnancy (as for clostridia). It is sometimes useful to establish whether there is an association with a particular field, season or age group and apply measures selectively.

Post-dipping lameness

Erysipelothrix can also invade broken skin. At the time of dipping, the organism from the soil can seriously contaminate the dip and enter limb wounds caused by handling at this time; within a day or so, many sheep may be very lame with a local cellulitis of the hairy parts of the limbs. Early treatment with penicillin is essential and, in future, ensure that dips are replenished regularly according to directions and that the tank is cleaned out.

Lambs up to 4 months - hill

Following tick bites and staphylococcal septicaemia (see page 79).

Old Ewes

A chronic degenerative arthritis of one or more joints, particularly elbows, shoulders, hips and stifles is quite often seen in elderly sheep (and shepherds!). They become progressively more lame and thin and need very careful attention. Culling (or retirement!) should be advised.

NUTRITIONAL MUSCULAR DYSTROPHY (NMD)

(Vitamin E and Se Deficiency (VESD),White Muscle Disease (WMD), Stiff Lamb Disease)

This is essentially a disease of young lambs which is becoming more common as a result of changing husbandry and feeding. Deficiency of either Vit.E or Se or both, causes sudden muscle weakness and lameness and sometimes sudden death in otherwise healthy lambs. The increasing tendency to feed only home-grown foods, to add preservatives to straw and cereals and to artificially fertilise with high N and SO_4, promoting rapid grass growth, have all led to overt clinical disease now appearing in areas which, as judged by river-bed surveys, have been short of Se for a long time.

Fortunately, the Se-responsive ill-thrift in lambs reported in other countries and the early foetal death leading to barren ewes and the increased susceptibility to disease because of reduced phagocytic activity, have not been confirmed in the United Kingdom.

Clinical signs

The usual story is that thriving young lambs (50% occur at 0–30 days and 25% at 30–60 days old) have just been turned out to fresh spring grass and within a few hours or days of running around, a few are found down and reluctant to get up; one or two may also be found dead due to cardiac failure. Those that are able to stand if forced to get up (you or your dog need to go into the field to find this out), take a few tottering steps and lie down again, looking alert and comfortable. Some may show distressed respiration due to failure of respiratory or cardiac muscles, and pneumonia is a secondary risk. This situation is, at first, easily confused with pulpy kidney, pasteurellosis, swayback, polyarthritis, spinal abscess and injury.

Diagnosis

(1) Suspicion arises if there has been previous evidence of Se deficiency on the farm and, in particular, if the flock is receiving little concentrate and no vitamin/mineral supplement and also if a lot of roots and/or poor quality roughage is being fed.

(2) The sudden onset in several otherwise healthy looking lambs should point to NMD and the absence of obvious signs of injury and arthritis should increase the suspicion.

(3) Necropsy should eliminate pulpy kidney disease and pasteurellosis, but note that the muscle lesions are bilateral and therefore no comparisons are possible within the lamb (you need to be able to visualise what you are looking for!) and that if there is cardiac involvement, the lungs may look pneumonic.

(4) Plasma and whole blood (green tubes) from affected lambs – plasma creatine kinase (CK) over 1,000 I.U./l = severe muscle damage, but the blood must be taken very early, as concentrations drop in a few days; whole blood glutathione peroxidase (GSHPx) often < 1 unit/ml.

(5) Whole blood (green tubes) from 10 apparently healthy contacts – GSHPx < 20 units/ml is suspiciously low.

(6) Inject with Vit. E and Se and see what happens!

Treatment

(1) Inject with Vit.E and Se (e.g. 1ml Dystosel - Intervet UK Ltd, costing approx. 35p) and repeat next day if not much improved. Usually there is a good (diagnostic) response if caught early.

(2) Rest – bring in.

(3) I/v methylene blue (1% solution) – 1ml/4.5kg body weight.

Prevention

(1) Ensure adequate levels of Se and Vit.E in the diet of ewes in late pregnancy:

(a) Avoid low Se foods, e.g. turnip and feeds which reduce Vit.E concentrations, e.g. treated grain, spoilt hay, oil seeds.

(b) Mineral/Vit. mix containing 15mg of Se and 1,500 I.U. of Vit. E per kg added to the concentrate at the usual rate of 25kg/tonne.

(2) Inject ewes once or twice in late pregnancy (e.g. Dystosel – Intervet UK Ltd, 2–3ml, costing up to £1.00).

(3) Various drenches (e.g. Panacur SC– Hoechst Animal Health; Pardevet– Bayer UK Ltd). These tend to be an expensive and inaccurate way of dealing with the problem, and risk Se toxicity if mis-diagnosed.

(4) Short-term control in lambs can be achieved by injecting them at strategic times, such as shortly before turnout or folding on roots (eg. Dystosel - Intervet UK Ltd, 0.5–1.0ml).

(5) Long-term control by:

(a) An annual injection to lambs at weaning and to pregnant ewes, of a long-acting barium-complex of Se (e.g. Deposel– Rycovet Ltd, costing 20–80p).

(b) Dosing weaned lambs and ewes once every three years with long-acting pellets (e.g. Permasel S – Coopers Pitman-Moore, costing approx. £1.50).

(c) In drinking water as sachets, e.g. Aquatrace, needing a piped water supply and preferably in troughs.

These long-term measures have not yet been properly evaluated in this country.

FOOT AND MOUTH (F & M) DISEASE

Fortunately, through lack of contact, this is likely to remain a rarity in sheep in the UK. It seems unlikely that F & M will arise as a primary outbreak in sheep because they are unlikely to be fed imported unsterilised meat. This means that practitioners will only be on the look-out for F & M in sheep in their area, following known outbreaks in other species.

F & M in sheep can present considerable problems, both because of the great difficulties in collecting and examining all the sheep in a flock and because sheep are known to act as carriers for several months.

Clinical findings

(1) Although the disease can be very mild in sheep, most people report systemic illness, with the sheep separated from the rest of the flock, looking unwell and unwilling to walk. (If you cannot catch the sheep, it is not F & M ??)

(2) Lameness, usually in more than one leg, is the most obvious feature. Early lesions are seen as blanching and separation of the interdigital skin at the coronary bands; after a day or so the lesions are ulcerative and granulomatous and easily confused with more common causes, e.g. early foot rot.

(3) Mouth lesions are less common and less severe and, therefore, sheep may eat and usually do not dribble frothy saliva as in cattle. If present, blanching and separation of the mucous membrane occurs, most commonly at the dental pad, which becomes ulcerated within a day or so of the initial blister.

(4) Ewes may abort and young lambs die (viraemia and myocarditis).

If you are in any doubt, ring the boss or the Ministry (for a diagnostic visit), *and stay on the farm*. If there are other stock on the farm enquire about lameness and examine.

LAMBING TIME

HOUSING EWES

Advantages

(1) Housing prevents damage to the pasture by the sheep, by poaching of land during the wet winter and by the nibbling of young grass shoots in February and March. This is particularly important on wet, heavy land and allows good grass growth in April when ewes are lactating heavily. This allows an increase in stocking rate which must follow housing if the costs are to be covered. Housing usually commences in December/January and sheep are turned out near the end of March, depending on weather.

(2) Housing improves the working conditions of the shepherd and protects sheep (and new-born lambs) from extreme weather conditions. Ewes are more carefully observed and shepherded during lambing which reduces lambing losses.

(3) Housing allows ewes to be sorted into different batches according to condition score, number of lambs being carried (if ultra sound pregnancy detection is used), state of teeth, lambing dates etc. and feed to be adjusted accordingly.

(4) Housing reduces the wastage of food if well-designed racks are used, whereas considerable wastage of concentrate occurs in adverse weather if fed outside. The feeding of the ewes is more controllable and regular condition scoring allows appropriate adjustment to feeding to be made.

(5) Housing allows (and usually necessitates) the shearing of ewes (see page 48).

Disadvantages

(1) Capital costs: These depend on the type of building and whether existing buildings can be modified. The building does not need to be of complex design but a purpose designed sheep house could cost up to £45 per ewe with an additional £5 for troughs. Much cheaper buildings are available, the cheapest being the 'polythene tunnel'. The latter building, composed of steel hoops covered with polythene and usually with walls of plastic mesh costs about £15–20 per ewe. The polythene covering has to be replaced periodically, some types every 3 or 4 years, but some last 10 years. Grants are no longer available towards the cost of housing and planning permission is needed if within 400 metres of residential buildings. Most buildings may be used for some other venture (e.g. calves) during the summer and autumn.

(2) Disease risks: Intensive housing may increase the risk of certain diseases such as neo-natal scours, coccidiosis, foot rot and pneumonia but these can be controlled by good construction and/or management.

(3) Food and bedding costs: Food costs in March will be increased because the young grass is deliberately not available to the ewes but this will be beneficial in the long run. Straw is an additional cost.

Principles of Design

Site

The house should be convenient for the shepherd, be sheltered from the prevailing wind and snow and have ready access to water and electricity.

Design

It is usual to have a wide centre passage, which may hold hay and concentrate feed and be used for lambing pens when the hay has been reduced. Pens to hold 30 – 60 ewes are sited on either side of the passage. The centre passage should be concreted but hardcore is best for the pens to permit good drainage.The size of pens varies with breeds and shearing but is about 1.0 - 1.3 sq. metres (10 - 14 sq. ft.) per ewe. It is most important that the ewe have ample trough space (0.45m/ 18 inches each). A useful design is to have removable, double-sided pen dividers consisting of a lower food trough and upper hay rack with a walkway along the middle of the rack. Straw bedding should be provided or slatted floors. About 2 bales of straw are needed for each ewe for a 3 month period.The house must be well ventilated above the sheep by Yorkshire boarding, plastic mesh, or open sides but be draught-proof at sheep level by having solid walls to a height of 1.0–1.2m. (3ft 3ins–4ft). Water may be provided in troughs, self-fill bowls or continuous flow along rainwater gutter. The water should be at a height that the sheep can reach but not too low or it will become contaminated with faeces and thought should be given to the increase in bedding height which occurs during housing. Good lighting is essential; artificial light should be 4 watts/sq. metre of floor space. Power points are also essential, for shearing and particularly for infra-red lamps over the individual lambing pens and for the shepherd's kettle! [Information on housing design and use of slats may be obtained from: Farm Buildings Information Centre, National Agriculture Centre, Stoneleigh, Kenilworth, Warwicks. CV8 2LG.]

SHEARING HOUSED EWES

Advantages

(1) It promotes a drier and cooler environment, with less heat stress in the ewes which therefore appear more comfortable.

(2) There are fewer disease problems associated with humid conditions eg. pneumonia, foot rot and lumpy wool.

(3) Ewes take less space, including trough space and more can be kept in a pen (up to 20%).

(4) Ewes eat more (if it is supplied!).

(5) Birthweight of lambs is increased and there are fewer cases of pregnancy toxaemia (if 4 applied).

(6) Thin ewes can be spotted easily and action taken (but very thin ewes should not be shorn).

(7) Ewes are cleaner and 'hung' lambs easier to see, promoting better lambing conditions for ewe, lambs and shepherd.

(8) The quality of shorn fleece is improved.

(9) There are fewer problems with lice and keds.

(10) Ewes are easier to blood sample.

Disadvantages

(1) Good housing is necessary if the sheep are not to become too cold and huddle together.

(2) Sometimes turn-out in the spring has to be delayed because of bad weather, leading to problems with housed lambs, bedding, feet and food costs. (At least 2 months' wool growth should be allowed before turn-out.)

(3) They are sometimes too hot in the summer with six months growth of fleece.

(4) There are increased feed costs.

(5) Single lambs may be too large, causing dystocia.

(6) 'Wool-Slip' – some wool loss is often noticeable in a proportion of the ewes. Various reasons have been suggested but the most likely appears to be that the dual stress of housing followed a few days later by shearing causes increased blood steroid concentrations, which is known to cause wool loss.

(7) The skin is more easily injured and infections, such as ringworm and staphs., become more widespread.

(8) There is a loss of quantity of fleece in the first year.

(9) Ewes are more difficult to catch, although they should not really be caught by the fleece (!) – and to truss.

CLOSTRIDIAL DISEASES

Clostridial diseases, other than tetanus, generally cause rapid death, therefore the practitioner is really only concerned with the problems associated with diagnosis and control. They are an ever-present risk.

Clostridial infections

Disease		Clostridium Sp	Age	Season	Trigger factors
1	Lamb dysentery	perfringens/welchii B	<2 weeks	spring	flush of milk
2	Struck	perfringens/welchii C	<2 weeks+adults	spring	flush of milk or grass
3	Pulpy kidney	perfringens/welchii D	>2 weeks	any	flush of milk, grass or concentrates
4	Tetanus	tetani	2–4 weeks	spring	docking/ castrating
5	Braxy	septicum	4–8 months	autumn	frosted food
6	Black	novyi/oedematiens B	adults	winter	fluke
7	Bacillary haemoglobinuria	novyi/oedematiens D	adults	winter	fluke
8	Blackleg post-partum gas gangrene malignant oedema	chauvoei, septicum	any	any	injury/wounds

Diagnosis

This needs to be speedy if control is to be effective. It is usually dependent upon obtaining from the farmer, accurate and relevant historical information (one is looking for a reason for the disease) supported, where possible, by post-mortem examination (PME) of fresh carcases. It is important not to rely on PME alone, not least because the material is often too decomposed for useful interpretation.

The information you need is:

(1) Did the sheep die 'suddenly'? (found dead).

(2) Were there any signs? (scouring, convulsions, stiffness).

(3) What age? (note the age ranges for the different clostridial diseases).

(4) What has the farmer done to control clostridial diseases? Have vaccines and/or antisera been used? (if so, closely check what and when).

(5) What has the farmer done to excite or introduce the disease? (e.g. change to better pasture or more concentrate, inject with dirty needles or irritant material, used rubber rings).

(6) Has the disease occurred on the farm before? (e.g. Lamb dysentery, Black).

(7) What season is it? (spring grass excites pulpy kidney and struck, fluke in winter excites Black, frost in autumn excites braxy).

(8) Are the affected sheep in good condition? (clostridial diseases often 'select' the greedy, fatter animals).

(9) Post mortem examination.

Control

Clostridial vaccines are so potent, so cheap and so available, it is not unreasonable to expect very few losses from clostridial diseases. However,VI centre reports continue to show that serious losses still occur (454 incidents in 1987) and that these are usually due to mistakes in application e.g. choosing the wrong mixture, injecting at wrong times, omitting injections and 'dirty' injections. Slick and clean s/c injection technique is needed to avoid abscess formation, in the neck site. The vet has a significant part to play in this area.

The recipe for control contains three ingredients:

(1) *Avoid the exciting factors*: In practice, this really means the control of fascioliasis, the use of sterile instruments and working in clean, dry conditions with dry, clean sheep.

(2) *Antibiotic cover* (e.g. long-acting antibiotic) following trauma, e.g. assisted lambing, dog bites.

(3) *Antibodies* derived via vaccination, colostrum or antisera.

Vaccination: There are a number of vaccines (e.g. Covexin 8, Tasvax 8) which protect against all the important clostridia. By using an 8 in 1 vaccine and efficient primary and secondary doses, it is possible to maintain a protective level of immunity throughout the year in both ewes and lambs, against all the usual clostridial diseases. Some other vaccines contain fewer antigens and may be cheaper, but it is arguably better to have a fully comprehensive insurance policy for these killing diseases. However, 7 in 1 vaccines are much used (omitting *Cl. novyi/oedematiens D*), and with 'Heptavac P' (Hoechst Animal Health) clostridial protection is combined with pasteurella. In Nilvax (Coopers Pitman-Moore), an 8 in 1 clostridial vaccine is combined with the anthelmintic levamisole; this is arguably an expensive way of dealing with the clostridial problem and often means underdosing and/or mistiming for worm control.

Two doses of vaccine at 6 weeks interval costing approximately 15p/dose, produce sufficient antibodies to protect a ewe for the first year with sufficient spare, via colostrum, to protect its lamb(s) for up to 16 weeks, providing the secondary or booster dose is given approximately 1 month before lambing. In subsequent years, only one pre-lambing booster injection is required to protect both ewe and lamb(s).

Assuming a flock to have no initial protection, one effective vaccination schedule is:

(a) *Ewes*

(i) Primary

(ii) Secondary - 6 weeks later

(iii) Booster - 2–4 weeks before lambing ((ii) and (iii) can be combined)

(iv) Repeat (iii) annually

(b) *Lambs* (ewe and ram)

Those to be kept over 16 weeks (for slaughter or breeding)

(i) Primary - at 12 weeks

(ii) Secondary - at 18 weeks

(iii) Booster (for breeding lambs only) at flock pre-lambing time (along with the adult ewes and rams)

(c) *Bought in ewes* (for tupping) *and store lambs* (for slaughter)

It is usually best to assume that these have not been vaccinated, or at least that their immunity has waned and to inject them 2 or 3 times in the first winter. A short-cut is often taken in the bought-in ewes (with some justification if there are no obvious winter clostridial risks, e.g. Black) and that is to vaccinate them on arrival but delay the secondary injection until 4 weeks before lambing.

(d) *Bought in rams*

If their vaccination status is in doubt, give 2 doses at 6 weeks' interval, followed by an annual booster.

(e) *Lambs out of unvaccinated or inadequately vaccinated ewes*

EITHER

(i) Primary – in first week, togetherwith Lamb Dysentery (LD) antisera if LD is a known risk.

(ii) Secondary - at 6 weeks.

OR

Rely on 200ml of colostrum (fresh or frozen) taken from a vaccinated ewe (or cow) and given at birth.

It is important to note that apart from the avoidable mistakes that some farmers make, it sometimes proves to be particularly inconvenient or impossible to inject sheep at the right times (particularly the pre-lambing booster) and also that not all lambs, particularly multiples, obtain adequate colostrum. The vet should be aware of such events on his clients' farms and advise accordingly, in particular, to ensure an adequate supply of frozen colostrum pre-lambing.

Cow colostrum is now very fashionable as a replacement for ewe colostrum. If good quality material is used (the first milking and before the calf is allowed to suck), it is clearly an adequate substitute food and most lambs tolerate it. To provide clostridial protection with cow colostrum, current work suggests that the cow can be vaccinated with sheep 8:1 vaccine (10ml 3 months before calving and again at 1 month and 2 weeks before calving) and 100ml of the subsequent colostrum (given by syringe or stomach tube) provides protection to the lamb for at least 3 months.

It is now known that, unfortunately, some cows produce a factor in their colostrum which, as the result of an immunological reaction, leads to the rapid removal of the recipient lambs' red cells together with the precursors in the bone marrow. This causes lambs about 10–14 days old to become suddenly and 'unaccountably' weak and to stop sucking; they show extreme pallor (PCV < 0.10) and they urgently require whole blood transfusion. This is most economically and conveniently supplied by taking blood from a ewe in a large syringe containing a drop of heparin, and giving it intraperitoneally (i/p 10ml/kg) as for glucose injection (see page 67). Valuable pedigree lambs may be given an orthodox transfusion. Corticosteroid and antibiotic injections are also indicated both to these lambs and to other lambs which may have received that batch of colostrum. A good response is expected within a day, although some die and reveal very watery blood and creamy white bone marrow on post-mortem examination.

It is important (although seldom practised!) to identify sources of colostrum, so that donating cows can be traced and problem ones avoided in future. Colostrum from goats is safer, providing it comes from Caprine Arthritis Encephalitis (CAE) accredited herds.

IN AN OUTBREAK, control measures in the rest of the flock consist of:

(a) Remove from the exciting source (where possible) e.g. take off the lush grass or reduce the concentrates.

(b) Antibiotic injection (e.g. penicillin) for those with local sepsis eg. 'gas gangrene' and tetanus.

(c) Antitoxin to all at risk , e.g. Lamb Dysentery, Pulpy Kidney, Tetanus.

As the protection provided by antitoxin persists for only approximately 2 weeks, it is appropriate to inject a primary dose of vaccine at the same time (but at a different site), followed by the secondary dose of vaccine 6 weeks later, thus providing both immediate and long-term cover; the potency of the antigen overcomes any significant interference by circulating antibody.

ABORTION

The incidence of abortions in 'normal' flocks is usually quite low (1 – 2%) and is usually tolerated by the farmer without investigation. However, it must be remembered that many of these abortions are caused by pathogens or nutritional disturbances, which also cause apparently 'barren' ewes, foetal mummies and very weak non-viable premature lambs. Abortions, therefore, should always be considered as only part of the losses in the production process and should be used as markers of what is often a much wider disease problem.

Example: In a 'normal' commercial lowland flock of 100 ewes, anticipating 180 live lambs, it is often true that up to 4 ewes will not produce lambs, 2 ewes will abort, and 20 lambs will be born either dead or die within a few hours of birth.

This means that the 100 ewes have only produced about 160 live lambs, and that about 10 of the ewes are 'unproductive'. In addition, probably 5 ewes will have died around lambing time for reasons not directly associated with abortions.

When, however, an abortion agent is introduced into a fully susceptible flock, the incidence of abortions is often alarming and is recognised as a 'storm'.

Causes

All abortions should be regarded as infectious until proved otherwise. The four most common causes of infectious abortion are:

(1) Enzootic (Chlamydial, EAE)

(2) Toxoplasma

(3) Campylobacter

(4) Salmonella – various serotypes

A number of other agents cause sporadic abortions:

Border Disease Virus

Listeria

Tick-borne fever – Rickettsia

Q fever – Coxiella

Corynebacterium pyogenes

Fungi

The confirmed prevalence of these infections varies with the area of the country and perhaps the interest of the laboratory.

The summary diagnoses reported from Veterinary Investigation Centres in England, Scotland and Wales in the Cumulate Diagnoses (VIDA II) for the years 1980–1987 inclusive give the following incidents of abortions in sheep (each a separate incident).

Abortion incidents reported by VI centres (1980-87)

	Number	%
Total abortion incidents	25567	100
Diagnosis not reached	12505	48.9
Chlamydia	5628	22.0
Toxoplasma	4301	16.8
Campylobacter	1235	4.8
Salmonellae	380	1.5
Other diagnoses	1518	5.9

Note the high percentage of incidents of abortions that are 'not diagnosed'. The most likely explanations for this are that laboratories:

(1) Often receive useless material.

(2) Can generally only consider infectious agents (and then perhaps only a few of these) .

(3) Receive just the 'odd' abortion from the 'normal' flock.

As a general rule, if there is a serious abortion problem and the laboratory receives sufficient useful material, the cause of abortion becomes apparent.

The diagnostic laboratory requires:

(1) Fresh foetal membranes with cotyledons (if these are not available then supply swabs from the wet skin of the foetus or of vaginal discharge.)

(2) Fresh foetus(es).

(3) Information, which will include:

Size and nature of flock, e.g. is it self-contained?

Are the abortions in a particular group, e.g. purchased, yearlings?

Feeding of flock.

Previous abortion history including any laboratory reports.

Dates of lambing.

Facilities for isolation.

Possible reasons for the abortion(s), e.g. handling and dosing, predisposing diseases, e.g. fluke and pregnancy toxaemia and dogs (though the evidence for the latter is very slight!)

(4) Blood sample for serum (red tube) for antibody for Toxoplasma or EAE (it is worth tagging aborting ewes so that they can be identified later).

Remember that some ewes can produce twins, one of which is apparently normal, and the other abnormal and infected. A flock may be infected with more than one pathogen, e.g. Toxoplasma and enzootic, so that it is worth continuing to submit aborted material to the VIC even after the first positive diagnosis has been established (perhaps 10% of subsequent abortions).

General Advice

Isolate aborting ewe and retain foetus(es) and membranes; treat as infectious (use poly glove and bags), not forgetting the public health risks from:

Chlamydia
Toxoplasma
Salmonella
Listeria
Q Fever

Toxoplasma and Chlamydia are particularly dangerous for pregnant women and their unborn children and they should not be involved with the lambing flock. Keep aborting ewes in isolation until a positive diagnosis has been made and until obvious vaginal discharge has ceased (up to 3 weeks) and tag so they may be identified later, if necessary, for blood or culling. If the ewe is ill, antibiotic therapy should be given but only after vaginal swabs have been obtained to submit to the laboratory.

Do not use aborting ewes or ewes producing premature lambs as foster mothers until it is known to be safe to do so.

It is usually better to retain aborting ewes and not sell them, because you hope that they will be now immune to at least one pathogen and not abort again.

The laboratory findings, e.g. Campylobacter, may suggest that it is a good plan to allow the aborted carrier ewe to mix with the ewes and lambs which have already lambed, and so induce general flock immunity,i.e.'move on' rather than'move back'. It is essential, however, to be absolutely certain that EAE is not also present before recommending this practice.

Bought-in sheep should mix with the resident sheep, general farm environment and on-the-farm food for as long as possible (3 months) before tupping, but they should, where possible, lamb separately in their first season on the farm, in case they are infected with Chlamydia and introduce EAE into the whole flock.

An abortion storm is usually not repeated in subsequent seasons and subsequent fertility is good, unless a different pathogen is introduced.

At the time of abortions, those ewes yet to lamb should be kept apart from the infected group and spread out, and the possibility of therapy (see specific infections) should be considered. Where possible, they should not lamb in the same area as the infected group, or at least the lambing yard should be re-strawed.

Enzootic Abortion (EAE)

This form of abortion is the most commonly diagnosed in the UK and is caused by *Chlamydia psittaci*, a highly specialised bacterium which parasitises host cells, in which it undergoes a complex life cycle involving the formation of reticulate and elementary bodies. *C.psittaci* has a very wide host range, including man, but different 'strains' exist and it is possible that some of these should really be regarded as separate species.

Although chlamydia are bacteria and are susceptible to certain antibiotics, they require 'virological' (tissue-culture) techniques for their isolation and propagation and cultural confirmation of diagnosis is not routinely available.

Infection of pregnant women causes death of the foetus and abortion and a very serious life-threatening disease in the mother.

Clinical picture

'Abortion' occurs in the last 2 or 3 weeks of pregnancy with no evidence of illness in the ewes. The pathology of infection is essentially a necrotic placentitis so lambs usually appear fresh and show little or no gross pathology, although the abdomen is sometimes distended with blood-stained fluid. In addition to aborted foetuses, premature and weakly live lambs, and even apparently healthy lambs but with infected membranes, are seen. Foetal membranes are sometimes retained, which may lead to metritis, but usually no clinical signs are seen in the ewes.

Epidemiology

(1) The most important source of infection is from aborting ewes since the organism is mainly excreted at the time of abortion and in subsequent vaginal discharges, which resolve in a maximum of 3 weeks. Infection is, therefore, mainly spread at lambing time and the rate of infection and the development of flock immunity is usually slow. Few 'storms' occur but the incidence of abortions tends to persist for years unless otherwise controlled. The disease is almost unknown in hill flocks where the management at lambing is less intensive than lowland, whereas it represents a serious and apparently increasing hazard for sheep lambing under intensive, housed conditions.

(2) Infection is introduced to a 'clean' farm by the purchase of ewes, which have usually lambed at least once, which are latently infected. The chlamydia are mobilised during pregnancy, giving rise to abortions etc. one year after the ewe became infected. No serological response can be detected during the 'latent' infection and there is no practicable method of deciding whether purchased ewes are infected. Since only a few purchased ewes may be infected and abort, material may not be submitted for diagnosis and the disease is not recognised until a much greater number of ewes abort at the next lambing season.

The characteristic picture, therefore, is that the first season of infection shows itself as a few purchased ewes aborting or producing premature lambs; the next one or two seasons, abortions and still-births occur in all age groups and the following seasons abortions etc are mainly confined to yearlings and bought-in sheep, since the older ewes will have acquired immunity, which is dependent on infection of membranes.

(3) Lambs can be infected at birth from their mother or other ewes and often produce infected lambs and membranes at their first lambing (which may not be until they are shearlings) and then become solidly immune.

(4) Ewes infected for the first time in late pregnancy do not usually abort then but may do at their next pregnancy. It takes about 40–50 days from infection to abortion which means that infection and abortion can occur within the same lambing season if batch lambing is practised. Ewes with lambing dates of more than 6 weeks apart should not be mixed close to lambing.

(5) Intestinal 'strains' of *C.psittaci* are common in sheep but their epidemiological significance is not known.

(6) Rams can become infected and may show epididymitis, but it is generally accepted that there is little likelihood that infection will be introduced into a flock or transmitted within a flock by rams. However, it seems unwise to purchase rams from flocks which are known to be infected.

(7) Recent studies indicate that chlamydia are not transmitted in the milk of infected ewes.

Diagnosis

There is usually an obvious placentitis with thickening and necrosis, so look at them before sending to VIC. Modified Ziehl-Neelsen staining of smears from the infected cotyledons shows intracellular inclusion bodies. However, infection may not be very obvious in the placenta when organisms are few and tissue culture has revealed organisms where smears have been negative. If no membranes are available, smears can be made from the wet skin/fleece of a recently aborted foetus or from the vagina of the ewe for 24 hours or so after abortion. Examination of the sera of an aborting ewe for complement-fixing (CF) antibodies will usually show a titre of at least 64 if EAE was responsible, but it is not usually necessary unless membrane material is not available. Interpretation of CF titres must take account of vaccination history and previous abortions because these may produce persistent titres.

Treatment

Aborting ewes rarely require any treatment other than isolation until their discharges cease. It is wrong to mix these with lambed ewes until discharges cease since the lambed ewes may become latently infected and abort next year.

A decision has to be taken immediately after a positive diagnosis has been made as to whether it is worth treating the ewes yet to lamb. This decision will be influenced by the size and value of the flock as well as a guess as to what the subsequent abortion incidence is likely to be! Oxytetracycline is effective against chlamydia and injection of a long-acting preparation (e.g. Terramycin/LA Injectable Solution, Pfizer Ltd, 20 mg kg i/m) will maintain pregnancy until nearer the expected lambing date. Injection could be repeated 2 weeks later for ewes which appear not to be close to lambing. Oxytetracycline does not sterilise the infection so membranes are still infective. Despite treatment, some ewes may abort or produce weak lambs and it is as well to warn the farmer of this fact.

In the first year after an outbreak in a valuable flock, it may be worth injecting oxytetracycline 3 and 6 weeks prior to the expected lambing date to reduce abortions in ewes which are latently infected.

Control

A. If EAE has been diagnosed, the following measures should be employed:

(1) Reduce transmission to other ewes.

(a) Remove and destroy all membranes, whether believed infected or not, by burial or burning.

(b) Attempt to clean up the area in the lambing shed and cover with clean straw.

(c) The use of aborted ewes to foster lambs should be discouraged but, if practised, the lambs must be sent for slaughter and females not retained for breeding since it is highly probable that they will have become latently infected.

(d) If there are only a small number of aborted ewes, they could be culled since some may continue to shed chlamydia, but if they are many, they may be kept as a basis of an immune flock.

(2) Protection of ewes by vaccination.

There is, at present, only one commercially produced vaccine in the UK. This consists of inactivated chlamydia from infected yolk sacs (Ovine Enzootic Abortion Vaccine (improved), Coopers Pitman-Moore, costing approx £2.50 a dose) and recommended to be given to all breeding females in late summer or early autumn before tupping, with revaccination 3 years later. Most farmers only vaccinate ewes once in their life, when they enter the flock. Vaccinating ewes and gimmers which had been orally infected the previous lambing season (i.e. the latent carriers) may prevent uterine infection, although it will not give 100% protection, and therefore the farmer should be warned that some of them might abort or produce weak lambs. In an emergency, the vaccine can be given to pregnant ewes exposed to infection in an attempt to prevent further abortions and/or infections, but it takes two months for neutralising antibody to develop, so the vaccine is only likely to have 'curative' value in those ewes more than two months off lambing.

There are sound reasons for vaccinating more frequently than every 3 years, especially since challenge is so high in housed sheep. In recent years, there have been abortions caused by chlamydia in ewes on farms where a proper vaccination programme has been used for many years. The vaccine has been modified to include a second strain of chlamydia and the number of reports of apparent breakdowns is now very small. They may be due to very heavy challenge, very virulent strains or antigenic differences. No reliable method is yet available to distinguish 'strains'. Infected membranes still occur in vaccinated infected ewes and infection is thus perpetuated on the farm.

B. If EAE is not present on the farm, strenuous efforts should be made to prevent its introduction:

(1) Maintain a self-contained flock. Rams may be purchased with little risk, but no female breeding stock or lambs for fostering should be purchased except from known clean flocks.

(2) Purchase replacements from flocks which are monitored free from EAE as part of the MAFF Sheep and Goat Health Scheme, the Premium Health Scheme for Sheep of the Scottish Agricultural Colleges or on other well-attested evidence.

(3) Lamb purchased ewes separately from the 'home' flock for the first year and investigate all abortions and apparently barren ewes, carefully.

Further reading

Aitken, I D (1986). 'Update : Chlamydial abortion in sheep', *In Practice*, Vol. 8, 236–37.

Buxton, D (1986). 'Potential danger to pregnant women of *Chlamydia psittaci* from sheep', *Veterinary Record*, Vol. 118, 510–11

Aitken, I.D., Clarkson, M.J. and Linklater, K (1990). 'Enzootic abortion of ewes', *Veterinary Record*, Vol. 126, 136-38.

Toxoplasmosis

Caused by *Toxoplasma gondii*, a coccidial protozoan, in which tissue cysts are found in virtually all mammals including man, and in birds, and in which a sexual cycle is completed only in cats and other Felidae, to produce resistant oocysts. When susceptible sheep ingest sporulated oocysts (*Toxoplasma* resemble *Isospora* oocysts, with 2 sporocysts each containing 4 sporozoites), the sporozoites penetrate the epithelial cells of the small intestine and are distributed to many organs, including muscles, brain and placenta in pregnant ewes. Multiplication occurs and cysts develop in these sites, which remain viable for the life of the sheep but are not mobilised. This means that adverse effects are only seen in pregnant ewes soon after the ingestion of oocysts. A solid immunity develops about 4 weeks after infection which lasts for life.

Infection of pregnant women by oocysts or from tissue cysts in undercooked meat may result in abortion or foetal abnormalities including hydrocephalus.

Clinical picture

This depends on the stage of gestation at which infection takes place. If oocysts are ingested in the first 60 days, foetal resorption occurs and the ewes may then appear to be barren, if the rams have been removed. Infection between days 60–120 results in the typical signs–abortion in late pregnancy, often with mummification of one or more foetuses, or with one or more stillborn lambs, or the production of weakly lambs. Infection after day 120 results in an infected normal lamb which becomes immune.

The ewes are not obviously ill, though they do have an increased temperature and lose appetite a few days after infection.

Epidemiology

(1) Sheep become infected by oocysts passed in cat faeces. Infection and abortion can result from infection with as few as 200 oocysts. The most likely sources of infection to sheep are by contamination of stored grain or hay or from pasture, by the spreading of manure containing cat faeces or by cats defaecating on the pasture. The oocysts are very resistant and remain viable for many months.

(2) Immunity following infection is strong and ewes never abort more than once. If infection occurs outside pregnancy, the ewe will become immune, without showing any signs.

(3) Although it is known that rams can excrete the organism in their semen for a short time after infection, this does not seem to be of importance and infection at this time, of course, would not result in abortion.

(4) Sheep to sheep transmission does not occur.

(5) Young cats become infected when they commence to hunt, particularly from mice and shed millions of oocysts over a few days about a week later.

Diagnosis

(1) Fresh foetal cotyledons often show small (2mm) white necrotic or calcified foci - 'White Spot Placenta' or 'Frosted Strawberries', often attached to brown, dry mummifying foetuses. The white foci are often easier to see if a microscope slide is placed on the cotyledon, or the cotyledon pressed against the side of a clear poly bag.

(2) Immunofluorescent antibody techniques on sections or smears of cotyledons may show brightly fluorescing tachyzoites or cysts.

(3) Serology on pleural or peritoneal fluids of still born lambs, live lambs *before* they have taken colostrum or *IgM* antibody in post-colostral live lambs. The presence of antibody in the foetus indicates an active infection in the uterus at the dangerous time.

(4) Histology or smears of placenta and histology or squash preparation of foetal brain may show Toxoplasma cysts or a specific cell reaction.

(5) Transmission of ground portions of placenta and foetus into mice. This takes up to eight weeks and, therefore, is only of use retrospectively.

(6) The detection of specific antibody by various techniques (e.g. indirect haemagglutination, latex agglutination, ELISA) is useful in epidemiological studies but antibody persists for years and serology is, therefore, of very little value in individual aborting sheep.

Treatment and Control

(1) During an outbreak of toxoplasmosis, aborting ewes are not dangerous to other ewes, or even useful in transferring infection and therefore immunity, so there is no obvious justification in continuing to isolate them once the diagnosis has been established. However, the farmer can easily become confused with this exception to the rule, and one must also always be aware of mixed infections, especially with chlamydia and zoonotic risks (handle abortions with care with disposable gloves).

(2) During the outbreak there is usually little to be done other than to grin and bear it, although it is prudent to look for the possible ways that sheep could have ingested cat faeces containing oocysts and postpone feeding any contaminated material until after lambing! Keep cats away from cereals, hay and bedding likely to be available to pregnant sheep (pelleted concentrate is likely to be safe).

(3) The organism is, however, susceptible to sulphonamides and injection (even one-off) of high dose trimethoprim and sulphadiazine (e.g. Tribrissen Injection 48%,Coopers Pitman-Moore at 60mg/kg (4 times the normal dose), costing approx £2.00 per ewe) is worth considering, although some foetuses will be dead and undergoing mummification at the time of treatment. One trial at Liverpool showed that treatment of half the ewes in a flock resulted in significantly more live lambs than in the untreated ewes. Unfortunately, pyrimethamine (Daraprim), a preparation used in man, cats and dogs for acute toxoplasmosis, is not easily absorbed via the rumen and is not useful for treating infected sheep.

(4) After lambing, retain the aborters and maintain within a closed flock, or introduce bought-in replacements to the farm environment, for as long as possible before tupping so that they are exposed to material likely to contain cat oocysts.

(5) A commercial vaccine has been produced in New Zealand which may be marketed in the UK soon. It consists of live attenuated tissue cysts and is injected into non-pregnant ewes. It is believed that it does not lead to tissue cysts in the ewes but stimulates a strong immunity.

(6) Chemoprophylaxis with monensin has proved effective in experimental and field studies in reducing the number of aborting and barren ewes. Monensin can be fed in a feedblock (Rumenco Ltd.) or in the concentrate, on veterinary prescription and ewes need to consume about 15mg per head per day. It must be fed continuously throughout pregnancy to control toxoplasmosis and is not 100% effective. Toxicity has been reported where the monensin premix was not mixed thoroughly with the concentrate.

It has been suggested that decoquinate (Deccox Sheep Premix, RMB Animal Health Ltd.) has a similar effect with less risk of toxicity, but this drug is much more expensive than monensin.

Further reading

Buxton, D (1989). 'Toxoplasmosis in sheep and other farm animals', *In Practice*, Vol. 11, 9–12.

Campylobacteriosis (Vibriosis)

Although the organism causing this form of sheep abortion was originally classified as *Vibrio fetus*, it is now agreed that it belongs to the genus *Campylobacter*. Sheep abortion is caused by *Campylobacter fetus* and *C. jejuni*.

(1) Infection is ingested, not venereal, and is primarily intestinal. It is therefore excreted in the faeces from symptomless carriers.

(2) Ewes are rarely ill at the time of abortion.

(3) Birds, e.g. crows and magpies, and voles may introduce the infection to a flock as well as introduced carrier sheep, and the infection is then spread from sheep to sheep via faeces, abortions and personnel.

(4) Early foetal loss is rare as ewes appear to be resistant in the first 3 months of pregnancy; campylobacter infection is therefore not associated with'barren ewes'. Bacteraemia follows infection in late pregnancy followed by placentitis which results in abortion 7–25 days after infection.

(5) Immunity following infection is strong to a particular serotype of which there are 3 in the UK, and subsequent fertility is good. Outbreaks may re-occur every few years because of lack of immunity in replacement stock, but usually abortions are few in number after the initial year of introduction.

Diagnosis

By smear and culture of cotyledons, foetal stomach or liver and visible focal necrosis of foetal liver is occasionally present. Campylobacter is not difficult to culture, but exact typing is complicated. Serology is not very helpful.

Treatment and Control

Usually the individual aborting ewe does not require any therapy. Once the diagnosis is confirmed, such ewes should mix with the ewes which have already lambed, but not with the pregnant sheep.

The remaining pregnant sheep must be kept away from the infection as far as possible and spread out, although the number and spread of abortions may not make this possible. Where a 'storm' is apparent, consideration should be given to antibiotic treatment of groups of pregnant ewes, with, for example, penicillin and streptomycin for 2 days or long-acting oxytetracycline.

The farmer should consider keeping a closed flock, although infection can be introduced by birds. He should not sell the aborting ewes. If he does buy replacements, he should mix them with the resident flock for as long as possible before mid-pregnancy, but separate them in late pregnancy.

Effective vaccines are available in some countries but not in the UK.

Salmonellosis

One sheep-specific salmonella, *S.abortus ovis*, causes abortion as do a number of other less specific serotypes including *S.typhimurium*, *S. dublin* and *S.montevideo*. *S. abortus ovis* is now rarely reported in the UK. The clinical picture is similar, but some serotypes are much more pathogenic for ewes than others.

(1) Abortions occur mainly in the latter half of pregnancy, although apparently barren ewes may reflect earlier foetal loss.

(2) Except for *S.montevideo*, ewes are often ill at/or before the time of abortion: some scour, some die, some have an offensive smelling vaginal discharge for a week or more.

(3) Except for *S.montevideo*, lambs are often ill at birth or subsequently, and develop a fatal septicaemia or pneumonia.

(4) Symptomless carriers are found in both ewes and lambs.

(5) A measure of immunity to a particular serotype is apparently induced because it is uncommon for ewes to abort the next season.

Diagnosis

(1) Salmonella is usually easily cultured from membranes and foetus, providing faecal overgrowth is avoided (a possibility if only vaginal swabs are provided).

(2) Blood testing and rectal swabs provide very little worthwhile information for the practitioner.

Treatment and Control

Salmonella is frequently found to be sensitive to a range of antibiotics in vitro and theoretically treatment of individual sick animals is indicated and also carriers (which usually means the whole flock). In practice such treatment frequently fails to cure the sick or sterilise the carrier, and is expensive. Furazolidone (Neftin 200, Smith Kline Animal Health Ltd.) has been used both in feed and by hand dosing, but without proven value. Consideration must be given in any salmonella outbreak to the risks of infecting man, and to producing drug-resistant organisms.

The principal aim in the control should be to:

(1) Reduce the weight of infection by the isolation of aborting, scouring and sick sheep and by high dose therapy with furazolidone or long-acting oxytetracycline of such animals. e.g. 50kg ewe – 250mg of furazolidone orally twice daily for 3 days. A 20% premix is available which can be mixed in the food to give the above doses for 7 days.

(2) Prevent further infection of pregnant sheep, as far as possible, by keeping the aborting group (usually the nearest to term) separate from other groups yet to lamb.

(3) Upset the flock as little as possible and make sure food (hay or concentrate) is always available, particularly immediately following flock movement.

(4) Try and ensure that most of the flock becomes immunised after lambing by spread from carrier ewes to non-pregnant ewes, i.e. mix recovered aborters with ewes that have lambed.

(5) Avoid re-introduction of the disease from sources such as 'foreign' slurry, bought-in sheep and other grazing stock, and infected feed (including bird faeces). Attempts should be made to prevent birds, especially magpies, entering sheep houses and feeding from the sheep troughs.

Further reading
Linklater, K A (1979). 'Abortion in sheep', *In Practice*, Vol. 1, 30–33.

FARMER'S FIRST AID CUPBOARD

Lubricant (e.g. Lubrel, Arnolds Veterinary Products)

Arm-length poly gloves

Lambing cords and figure-of-eight telephone cable (or e.g. Hughes Lambing Snare, Arnolds Veterinary Products)

Lamb stomach-tube and syringe (e.g.'Arn-Lam' feeder, Arnolds Veterinary Products)

Frozen colostrum (200ml lots)

Antibiotic injection (e.g. LA oxytetracycline)

Antibiotic drench for lambs (e.g. Clamoxyl oral doser, Beecham Animal Health)

Ophthalmic antibiotic (e.g. Aureomycin ophthalmic, Cyanamid UK)

Glucose 20% injection (e.g. Dextrose 20, Bimeda UK Ltd.)

Calcium/Magnesium injection (400ml bottles of 20% Ca)

Oral glucose (Liquid Lectade, Beecham Animal Health)

Tincture of iodine (e.g. in a spray)

Cotton Wool

Spirit

Needles 16 x 1", 18 x 1/2", 19 x 1"

Syringes 50, 10 and 5ml

Thermometer (to test lamb for hypothermia)

SOME GYNAECOLOGICAL PROBLEMS NEAR PARTURITION

Vaginal prolapse (eversion of the vagina/cervix)

This is an important problem, the cause of which is still uncertain. The incidence, although generally low(1%), and very low in hill sheep, is sufficient to be a worry, and in some flocks over 5% of the ewes are affected and over a short period. Minor prolapses may not cause much disturbance, popping in and out as the ewe gets up and lies down, but if left, severe complications often arise which endanger both the ewe and the lambs; the condition must therefore always be taken seriously and treated quickly.

The prolapse usually occurs in the last 3 weeks, and particularly the last week, of pregnancy in ewes carrying more than one lamb. There is sometimes an association with a particular breeding line or breed of tup, and ewes that prolapse often do it again next year. Cases therefore need to be marked for culling, as well as to spot breed connections.

Many causes have been suggested including multiple lambs, condition of ewe (too fat or too thin!), gut-fill and roughage, calcium deficiency, hormone imbalance, short docking, steep ground and coughing!

The best control advice at present is to:

(1) Assess the ration; in particular the quality and quantity of the roughage in relation to the ewes' condition score and foetal load.

(2) Mark, *record* and cull cases.

(3) Consider these records and note susceptible lines and breeding.

Replacement of the prolapse,after cleaning up, is usually easy at first, but if there is delay, damage and subsequent swelling promotes further straining; it is then helpful to suspend the ewe and as the prolapse is returned, allow urine to flow from the occluded and distended bladder. The prolapse is then retained by one of three methods:

(1) Wool-tying – for only the simplest cases, and not applicable for shorn ewes!

(2) Vulval sutures - several techniques, but they all need removal at lambing if they don't tear out before!

(3) Truss- using

  (a) string, or for the more persistent cases, the webbing and leather Devonian Ewe Truss.

  (b) Wire or plastic intravaginal devices (e.g. Arnolds' Ewe Prolapse Retainer).

As complications are common, such as persistent straining, ringwomb and dead lambs, the ewe requires special observation. To reduce abdominal pressure, the quantity of roughage should be reduced and antibiotic cover provided where there is obvious mucosal damage; the caesar pack needs to be handy.

Vaginal Rupture/Intestinal Prolapse

This is probably a severe variation of vaginal prolapse, with the same background circumstances. A rupture of the vaginal wall occurs near the dorsum of the cervix with loops of intestine prolapsing through the vulva. Death is rapid.

Uterine Prolapse

This occurs usually immediately after lambing and the ewe is not obviously shocked. After cleaning up and removal of any foetal membranes, and with the ewe suspended, the uterus is usually easy to replace and to retain with truss/sutures. Some prolapses occur a few days after lambing, and then shock is often more serious and death is common.

Abdominal Rupture

This is again usually noticed in late pregnancy and in lowland ewes carrying twins or triplets. The rupture may involve any part of the abdominal wall and although the ewe is not usually distressed or disturbed at first, complications may arise from stricture of the contents, and it may interfere with lambing. Surgical correction is usually impossible but the caesar pack may be needed. Old ewes are most prone, particularly if they are too thin, and perhaps if they are squeezed or knocked during handling and housing.

Further reading
Hosie, B (1989). 'Vaginal prolapse and rupture in sheep', *In Practice*, Vol. 11, 215–18.

OBSTETRICS

It has been calculated that:

(1) 70% of ewe deaths occur at or near lambing.

(2) at least 75% of lamb deaths occur at or near lambing.

(3) 90% of vets' visits occur at or near lambing.

These figures demonstrate that parturition is a high risk occupation and also that vets are 'dangerously' dependent upon this time for their contact with sheep farmers; but it is rewarding work!

Uterine manipulation is relatively easy in most breeds, particularly for small hands, and limited embryotomy and caesarian operations are simple procedures.

There are particular problems associated with certain breeds and different problems in hill and lowland flocks.

The seasonal pattern of lambing presents problems, with sudden numbers and lack of practice, a large susceptible population and very intensive conditions.

Shepherd interference is the rule and the lamb(s) are often dead when the vet's assistance is sought. The shepherd's job is usually quite different to the vet's – the shepherd has a problem of numbers, timing (when to interfere), observation, cleanliness, and often very simple manipulations, principally the removal of 'tight' lambs in normal presentation and position, and to ensure the lambs are not smothered and/or mis-mothered.

Maternal factors

Ewes do not withstand prolonged vaginal and uterine interference; a sick ewe = a dead ewe!

Uterine, cervical and vaginal tears are common following rough handling and inadequate lubrication.

Clostridial sepsis is common after vaginal interference if vaccination is inadequate and/or antibiotic not injected.

Retention of the foetal membranes is rarely a problem.

Foetal factors

Often more than one lamb - a sorting out job - be patient.

Head and leg deflections common.

The head is the major cause of obstruction and there is rarely sufficient room in the pelvis for the lamb's head and legs plus your hand, so use a snare over the head to permit traction.

Tight lambings can cause hepatic and/or intra-cranial haemorrhage leading to rapid death, or recumbent and hypothermic lambs which need urgent attention.

Equipment

Lubricant and small hands.

Antibiotics: Parenteral, single-dose, long-acting antibiotic.

Snares: 3 braided cords or binder twine with one labelled. Figure-of-eight telephone cable to act as 'snare', or Hughes Lambing Snare (Arnolds Vet Products)

Sharp knife.

History

How long has the ewe been lambing? The normal range is approximately:

Change in temperament	2 to 4 hours
Cervical dilatation	1/2 to 2 hours
Delivery	1/2 to 2 hours

Have any lambs been born or delivered?

Examination

Take special note of the following:

External:

Does the ewe look ill or exhausted?

Are there signs of shepherd interference? Note bleeding and bruising.

Presence or absence of lamb/membranes at vulva.

Smell.Putrefaction implies bad risk,little value and embryotomy rather than caesar.

Udder. May indicate prematurity, mastitis, lack of colostrum.

Internal:

Ewe: The size and shape of the pelvis.

Any damage to the vagina.

The extent of softening and dilatation of the cervix. If the cervix is not fully dilated, re-examine in about 1/2 an hour, rather than risk manual dilation.

Lambs: Dead or alive? (not always easy to be certain assume alive if not sure)

How many?

Presentation/position?

Delivery

Aim to complete delivery within 15 minutes.

Lubrication very important.

Suspending the ewe can help to avoid straining and allow repulsion of a lamb.

Anterior presentation:

The head is the main bulk. It may require snaring. It is common for only a swollen head to be presented outside the vulva,with both front legs 'back'. If the lamb is dead (no suck or blink) then decapitate; if alive, then suspend the ewe, lubricate and insert a small hand beside the head and neck and try to find a limb and extend it. It is often then possible in ewes (but not ewe – lambs) to withdraw the lamb with only one limb extended.

Head and neck deflections are common- try finger grips in eye socket or mouth. Repulsion of limbs may be necessary with the ewe suspended but be careful because cervical and uterine tearing is easy; snare the limbs first.

Posterior presentation:

Provided both hind-limbs and tail are present, withdraw with gentle traction but beware of excess pressure on the lamb's rib cage causing hepatic rupture and fatal haemorrhage. Often only a tail is presented = breech, and again, some repulsion is necessary. Search for the hind legs of that lamb and bring them up one at a time into the pelvis by flexing/extending the limb joints.

Embryotomy:

This consists of simple decapitation or skinning and removal of limbs of a known dead lamb OUTSIDE the vulva, with just a sharp knife and fingers.

Caesarian Operation:

Indications:

(1) Non dilatation of cervix after 1 or 2 examinations at approx. 1/2 hour intervals.

(2) Foetal oversize.

(3) Irreversible mal-presentation.

(4) Deformities.

(5) Uterine torsion (very rare).

(6) Pregnancy toxaemia - rarely successful for lambs.

The operation is relatively quick and easy, compared with other species, and needs to be considered early in the proceedings rather than too late!

After Delivery

(1) Re-examine for:

(a) presence of other lamb(s)

(b damage

(c) membranes

(2) Antibiotic injection and intra-uterine pessary or powder.

(3) Udder.

(4) Attention to lamb(s).

Revival and survival – suspend, blow in nostrils, dry and warm, return to dam quickly for licking.

Colostrum – via dam or bank.

Navel – tincture of iodine spray or antibiotic aerosol.

NB Madel's rule for lambings = 1L + 4R'S = Lubrication, Recognition, Repulsion, Removal, Re-examination.

Further reading

Cox, J E (1987). *Surgery of the reproductive tract in large animals*, Liverpool University Press.

PERINATAL PROBLEMS

Many farmers accept that up to 15% of all lambs are either dead when born or die within the first few days of life (occasionally these losses rise to 50%, e.g. in abortion storms and seasonal sway-back). This means that in a flock of 1,000 lowland ewes anticipating 1,800 lambs, over 250 lambs may be lost in the perinatal period (0–10 days).

These losses can be split into:

(1) *Pre-partum stillbirths* (including abortions) –2%.

Many of these will be due to uterine infections such as Toxoplasma, Salmonellae, Campylobacter, Enzootic Abortion, Border Disease, plus Tick Borne Fever, Pregnancy Toxaemia and Swayback.

(2) *Parturient stillbirths* (dystocias) – 5%. If the losses are due mainly to lambing problems, then the quality and quantity of the workforce needs looking at, and also the age, breeding and feeding, e.g. large singles, and ewe-lambs that are CS4 and crossed with a Texel ram!

(3) *Post-partum mortality* – 8%

Often said to be born dead, but actually died soon after birth .

It is important to try and split lamb deaths into these three groups by fresh post-mortem examination, in order to apply sensible control measures, e.g. if the deaths are mainly pre-partum one has to look for causes of death in-utero; if at birth, then the shepherd's vigilance and availability may be inadequate; if after birth, then lambs have probably not sucked adequately and have become cold.

Post Mortem Features (on 'Fresh Neonates')

(1) Decomposition – indicates pre-partum death , as does clouding of cornea.

(2) Weight – singles 4.5kg; twins 3.5kg (allow for breed variations). Excessive weight suggests dystocia, underweight suggests a pre-partum problem, e.g. feeding of ewe or uterine infection.

(3) Umbilical vessels- arteries are empty if death is pre-partum/partum. A thrombus indicates that death is post-partum. The thrombus develops at the end of the umbilical arteries and propogates up the vessel. In lambs dying immediately before or during parturition, the end of the artery is sharply pointed, but if some time pre-partum, the ruptured end is square. The end is shrivelled if death is post-partum.

(4) Presence of food in stomach - indicates post-partum death.

(5) Lung aeration indicates partum or post-partum death.

(6) Subcutaneous oedema of distal legs/tail and head – indicates dystocia or hypothermia.

(7) Hepatic rupture, thoracic, abdominal and meningeal haemorrhage (open up cranium and spinal canal) - indicate dystocia.

(8) Fat-lambs are born with fat reserves (brown/yellow) which support it during the first few days of life. In starvation, as the fat is metabolised, it is replaced by soft, red gelatinous tissue.

(9) Wear on feet – indicates lamb has lived for a few hours.

Further reading

McFarlane, D (1965). 'Perinatal lamb losses: an autopsy method for investigation of perinatal losses', *New Zealand Veterinary Journal*, Vol. 13, 116–35.
Wilsmore, A J (1989). 'Birth injury and perinatal loss in lambs', *In Practice*, Vol. 11, 239–43

Early Post Partum Problems

It is well to remember that these are often an expression of PRE-PARTUM disturbances

e.g. so-called soft lambs	Enzootic abortion
hairy shakers	Border Disease
ataxia/paresis/ recumbency	Daft Lamb, Swayback and Muscular Dystrophy

and often indicate inadequate feeding of the ewe in late pregnancy, which leads to:

(1) Short gestations, giving small weak lambs with poor protective fleeces and little brown fat reserve. Such lambs become hypothermic and unable to rise. They require a bit of luck with the weather, and a good mothering shepherd, if they are to survive.

(2) Poor mothering and less colostrum and milk, less suckling and then, less sucking and a vicious circle. This not only leads to hypoglycaemia and hypothermia, but surviving lambs are more susceptible to post-partum infection because of the reduced colostrum intake.

(3) Specific deficiencies of copper and selenium leading to Swayback and Muscular Dystrophy.

In common with all other species, lambs are exposed to a variety of POST-PARTUM infections introduced orally, via the navel, or via docking and castration.

Oral	*Cl.perfringens B* (Lamb dysentery) *E.coli*- K99 enterotoxigenic (ETEC) strains. Salmonella – *S.typhimurium* and *S.dublin* the most common. Cryptosporidia Rotavirus Parapox virus (orf)
Navel	Staphs., Streps., *E.coli*, Fusiforms, Clostridia *C.pyogenes*.
Castration/docking	*Cl.tetani*

Such infections produce a variety of CLINICAL SIGNS such as:

Hyperexcitability, tremors, opisthotonus, nystagmus, convulsions, coma.

Dull, sleepy, weak, recumbent.
Salivation.
Atony of gut, with abdominal distension and no faeces.
Scour.
Navel Ill.
Joint Ill.
Ataxia/paresis.
Scabby lips and proliferative sores on gums and tongues.

However, farmers (and sometimes vets!) are inclined to place too much significance on these pathogens and therefore on therapy, whereas the main problem more often stems from susceptible lambs and/or weight of infection via dirty conditions, instruments and hands, as well as inadequate observation, isolation and treatment of individual cases. As a general rule, offspring survive if they are average birthweight, kept warm and receive adequate colostrum, whereas those that are small, cold and fail to obtain adequate colostrum, die.

Investigation of Perinatal Problems

It needs time and thought and should include:

(1) History –

Numbers involved (size of problem). Problems in previous years. Purchases and related incidence of disease (is the problem confined to one group? e.g. replacement ewe-lambs). Breeding and lambing dates. Weather conditions throughout pregnancy. Feeding of ewes, vaccination and dosings (e.g. copper, fluke). Farmer's account of mortality, clinical signs/ treatment.

(2) Farm observations –

Cleanliness, drugs and instruments, shelter, isolation and warmth, feed available including colostrum, (do your observations agree with the farm story?), shepherding quantity and quality.

(3) Clinical examinations –

Ewes - age, condition score, udders.
Weak lambs - age, size, clinical signs, castration/docking.

(4) Laboratory –

Plenty of fresh material(including foetal membranes). It may include paired blood samples from marked ewes for enzootic abortion, toxoplasma and Border Disease Virus, plus blood biochemistry (copper and GSHPx).

Some specific post-partum problems

Hypothermia

If a very young lamb is weak and with a temperature of less than 100°F (38°C) it requires firstly drying (if wet), preferably with a dry towel, then warming and feeding (warm colostrum if less than 12 h, or warm milk if over 12h). If it is collapsed and not able to sit up on sternum (but avoiding the watery mouth and scouring lamb), give it an intra-peritoneal injection (just below and to one side of the navel, with the lamb held up by its front legs) of 25–50ml of warm 20% glucose solution (Bimeda UK Ltd.) and parenteral antibiotic (e.g. 0.5ml Terramycin L.A. Injectable Solution, Pfizer Ltd.). When the lamb is conscious and able to suck, feed 150–200ml at least 3 times a day via bottle or stomach tube until the lamb is able to suck the ewe vigorously. If the lamb is one of twins, remove the other from the ewe and return them together when ready.

Warming a lamb is best done in a box with a domestic blower placed under a wire mesh floor.

Watery Mouth, Slavers, Rattle Belly

These are common terms used to describe a condition which affects very young lambs (up to 3 days old), characterised by the following:

(1) Lambs rapidly become dull and weak, look miserable and don't get up, and they become unwilling to suck.

(2) They have cold, wet lips and muzzles from drooling saliva, but note that terminally ill lambs dying of other causes often drool saliva.

(3) No faeces are visible (meconium) and the tail is dry.

(4) The temperature is at first normal, but hypothermia follows.

(5) The abdomen is relaxed at first and looks full, but later there is tympany and tenseness which causes 'rattling' when tapped or shaken, and the distension may cause distressed breathing.

(6) Without treatment, they usually die within the day, but some live long enough to develop scouring and even joint ill, just to complicate the picture!

(7) The incidence can be frighteningly high (>20%), and is most common in twins or triplets from ewes with condition score <3 and lambed indoors.

Cause

The current theory is that lambs which develop Watery Mouth have swallowed too little colostrum and too many non-ETEC *E.coli* in the first few hours of life, resulting in gut stasis and the absorption of bacterial endotoxins. This theory seems to fit most of the observed events and leads to a rational approach to effective treatment and control.

Treatment

(1) I/M and oral antibiotic against *E.coli* (e.g. Clamoxyl L.A. injection and Clamoxyl Oral Multidoser- Beecham Animal Health).

(2) 100–200ml of glucose/electrolyte solution (e.g. Liquid Lectade – Beecham Animal Health) by stomach tube three times a day until sucking.

(3) Warm soapy-water enema (10–20 ml via cut-down stomach tube).

(4) Leave the ewe and lamb(s) together, and keep warm.

Control

(1) Increase the colostral protection:

(a) Feed the ewes well so that CS is at least 3.

(b) Ensure good bonding (avoid moving ewe and lamb too soon after birth).

(c) Ensure the lamb(s) suck (avoid early castration and have good shepherding).

(2) Reduce the weight of infection:

(a) Keep things as clean as possible; bedding, pens, udders.

(b) At birth, oral dosing of lambs with a suitable antibiotic.

On farms with a history of high incidence, give all lambs, shortly after birth, 100–200ml of cow colostrum. Unfortunately, the current *E.coli* vaccine (Coliovac, Hoechst Animal Health) appears not to provide protection, and the ETEC *E.coli* K99 antigen does not appear to be involved in the condition.

Further reading
Eales, A and Small, J (1984). *Practical lambing*, Longman.
Eales, A (1987). 'Watery Mouth', *In Practice*, Vol. 9, 12–17.

Neo-natal Diarrhoea/Scours

Whilst individual scouring lambs can be dealt with without resort to laboratory diagnosis, it is important in an outbreak or in any flock with a persistent problem with scouring lambs to establish, if possible, if there is one dominating causal organism. To do this requires submitting up to 10 faeces samples (20–30ml, if possible), as well as any terminally ill untreated lambs and/or fresh carcases. This should provide sufficient information to prescribe appropriate treatment and control measures.

In the case of Lamb Dysentery, this will mean antisera to lambs at birth for this season, and for the next season a proper ewe vaccination policy. Salmonellosis will require special advice about the risk of spread to other species, including personnel, and the sero-typing and antibiotic sensitivity testing of *E. coli* will lead to an appraisal of vaccination (e.g. Coliovac, Hoechst Animal Health) and the choice of antibiotic. Treatment and control of Rotavirus and Cryptosporidia infections will have to rely on non-specific measures (clean pens, good colostrum intake, etc.).

In general, it is vital to provide isolation, warmth and plenty of fluids (e.g. Liquid Lectade, Beecham Animal Health) and when in doubt about the causal organism, to initiate antibiotic treatment aiming at *E. coli* (e.g. Clamoxyl Oral Multi Doser and Clamoxyl L.A. Injection, Beecham Animal Health).

Further reading
Mitchell, G and Linklater, K (1983). 'Differential diagnosis of scouring in lambs', *In Practice*, Vol. 5, 5–11.

Treatment of Navel and Joint – ill and lambs with CNS involvement

Vigorous and prolonged (7–14 days) systemic treatment with high dose, twice daily penetrating antibiotic (e.g. Trivetrin, Coopers Pitman-Moore, 0.5–1.0 ml). Flunixin and anti-convulsants may also be indicated and also joint perfusion.

General Control Measures

(1) Break in the lambing sequence (batch lambing).

(2) Cleanliness – instruments, hands, bedding and disposal of foetal membranes/carcases. Change lambing pens/areas (even re-strawing of area is helpful), turn out.

(3) Provision of adequate shelter (even a zig-zag of straw bales in the field is helpful).

(4) Reduce stocking density.

(5) Spraying navels with tincture of iodine.

(6) Early detection and isolation of cases.

(7) Ensure a good supply of frozen colostrum which can be obtained from donor ewes (give 1 ml oxytocin and wait 15 minutes) or cows (see page 51).

(8) Consider *E.coli* vaccination('Coliovac', Hoechst Animal Health), price approx 30p/dose. It has a schedule similar to clostridial vaccination and can be given simultaneously.

(9) Cull ewes that are thin and have faulty teeth and/or udders; feed the others properly.

(10) Review future policy for vaccination, feeding and the provision of copper and selenium.

MASTITIS

The 1983 edition of this handbook contained no section on mastitis because we felt that there was little useful to say to the clinician on the subject because of both lack of concern and good data. This is now changing and, thankfully, the pattern of disease is becoming better understood and control measures more authentic, although still a long way behind our knowledge of mastitis in the dairy cow (see *Mastitis Notes for the Dairy Practitioner*, Liverpool University Press 1987).

Two forms of the disease are apparent:

(1) Healthy ewe with chronic, palpable mastitis = grade 2C

(2) Sick ewe with acute, often gangrenous mastitis = grade 3

Both forms are irreversible, the first require culling and the second life-saving.

Chronic Mastitis (grade 2C)

This is usually discovered before tupping at a time when the ewes are selected for breeding or culling (e.g. thin, teeth, barren, known disease). One half of the udder, less commonly both, is lumpy and distorted with palpable chronic abscesses. The flock prevalence varies between 1% and 15%. If these cases are not spotted at this time, they become apparent at lambing and probably account for many of the ewes which lamb-down with only one functional gland, and for the problem of neo-natal disease that this invites. It is uncertain when infection occurs, but it is assumed that it is at weaning time, because long-acting antibiotic, introduced then, is known to reduce the disease incidence. This is very similar to the dairy cow story and the range of organisms appears to be much the same,with staphylococci the favourite.

Control is suggested in the following ways:

(1) Dry Ewe Therapy (DET) at weaning – with e.g., 1/2 tube of Streptopen DC (Coopers Pitman-Moore) or 1 tube of Orbenin DC (Beecham Animal Health) per gland. This is a two person job and the teats need to be cleaned before infusion.

(2) Place ewes on poor keep and reduced water at weaning and keep well away from the sound and sight of their lambs, to reduce milk production.

(3) It seems a reasonable idea to teat-dip with a commercial cow teat dip at the time of infusion.

(4) Colour tag cases for culling.

Acute Mastitis (grade 3)

This occurs most commonly early in lactation, when the ewe is milking well and being sucked fiercely. It seems that it sometimes follows movement onto lush clover pasture or a period of rough weather, and shorn or crutched ewes are perhaps particularly vulnerable shortly after turn-out. The clinical picture is dramatic and typical; the ewe is obviously ill with a swollen udder (usually only one half), she walks stiffly and the lambs appear hungry, the teat and a portion of the udder skin often become cyanotic and cold, and oedema extends along the region of the mammary vein. Slow sloughing often occurs if the ewe survives the first day or so, with an extensive loss of abdominal skin, leaving tubes of mammary ducts and blood vessels exposed. Healing then takes many weeks and the ewe loses much condition and it may be necessary to tie off and amputate these granulating tubes to speed healing and also to take measures to avoid fly-strike.

Staphylococci and *Pasteurella haemolytica* are the principal pathogens, but *Escherichia coli* and *Corynebacterium pyogenes* are also on the list, as well as, surprisingly, *Clostridium perfringens*. This range of organisims is interesting and hopeful because there are commercial *E. coli*, clostridia and pasteurella vaccines designed for use in pregnant ewes and staphs. and *C. pyogenes* are tailor-made for DET (compare the dairy cow). In addition, orf on ewes' teats after lambing is a significant hazard and vaccination at around tupping time might help to solve this problem.

Treatment

Vigorous systemic treatment is indicated as soon as a case is detected, but the local pathology is often already irreversible. High dose of an antibiotic which is likely to cover the range of bacteria is recommended (e.g. Trivetrin Injection, 3ml/50kg, Coopers Pitman-Moore), and repeat twice daily until the ewe shows improvement (a day or so) or dies! Strip the gland out each time the ewe is treated and drainage is aided by removal of the teat if gangrenous. Intra-mammary tubes are an optional extra. Ensure the ewe is comfortable, preferably in isolation, and has tempting food and water nearby. I/v fluids (1-2 litres) and flunixin are also indicated.

Control

This sporadic condition simulates the problem of grade 3 environmental mastitis in dairy cows, and its control is equally difficult. There is evidence that it does not arise from pre-existing sub-clinical intramammary infection, but from opportunistic invasion shortly before clinical events; this suggests that DET is unlikely to be effective.

The incidence varies between seasons, perhaps because of changing management and climate, but it is usually of the order of 1%; this level makes the condition of only nuisance order to the farmer and militates against whole-flock control measures.

Some suggestions:-

(1) If ewes are too thin (CS <3), consider increasing the feed and so ensure adequate milk for vigorous lambs.

(2) Attend to teat sores - pustules, orf and sucking wounds; this may mean antibiotic injections and even weaning the lamb(s).

(3) Avoid turning out in cold wet weather and/or ensure shelter.

(4) Clean, dry bedding at lambing ('Squelch' test!).

(5) Ensure proper clostridia vaccination and consider *E. coli*, pasteurella and orf vaccination for this and other reasons.

(6) DET and teat dip, if records/history show that cases occur at or very near lambing (consider a trial group if thought too expensive to do the flock).

(7) Colour tag cases for culling.

Swayback
Border disease
Daft lamb disease
Cerebro-cortical necrosis (CCN)

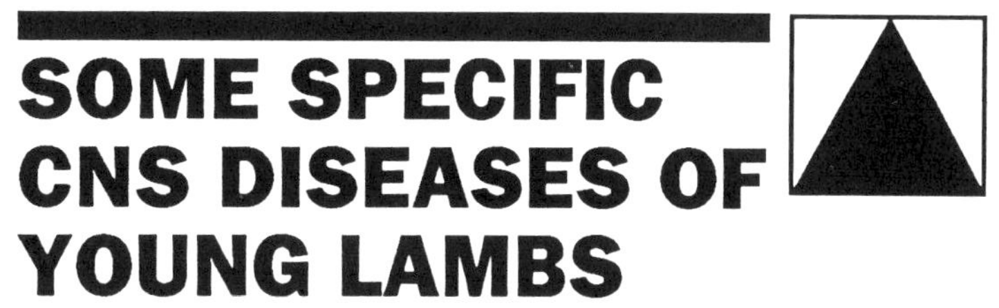

SOME SPECIFIC CNS DISEASES OF YOUNG LAMBS

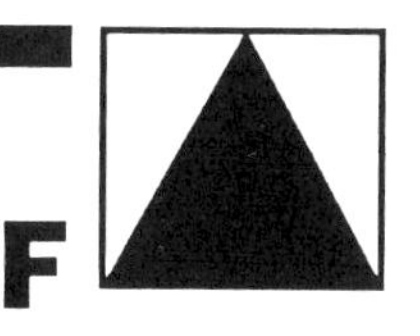

In addition to the CNS diseases of young lambs which may follow any post-partum bacteraemia or septicaemia, there are three specific conditions, Swayback, Border Disease and Daft Lamb Disease, which originate pre-partum. These need differentiation and whilst at first the clinical signs may appear non-specific or confusing, careful history taking and clinical examination should give you the confidence to arrive at a provisional diagnosis; this usually needs biochemical and histological support before flock control measures are introduced.

SOME QUESTIONS OF HISTORY

Ask the farmer to describe the clinical signs.

When did the signs first show? At birth, 1 week + etc.

How many cases have there been so far this season?

How many normal lambs are there?

How many have died?

Do any get better? – with or without treatment.

Are the affected lambs out of one particular batch of ewes?

Are they single lambs?

Has the farmer 'done anything' to them recently? – changed pasture, weaned, dock/castrate, inject/drench.

Has the farmer any cases which can be examined today?

Are there ticks?

Ask questions about the ewes – abortions, breeding, copper supplementation.

SWAYBACK (Enzootic Ataxia)

This is one of the most important of the many central nervous diseases of lambs, and is caused by faulty development and degeneration of nervous tissue in the brain and spinal cord of lambs whose mothers had low copper concentrations in the blood in the latter part of pregnancy.

These clinical notes assume a knowledge of the pathology and diagnostic clinical pathology of the condition, as well as the toxicology of copper. It is very important to remember that copper still heads the list of poisons in sheep (93 incidents in 1987 at VI Centres).

Diagnosis

(1) *History*: Suspicion arises from one or more of the following:

(a) Swayback has been diagnosed clinically on the farm before.

(b) Copper has not been given to the ewes during pregnancy.

(c) It has been a mild winter. This influences the quality and quantity of the grass, the amount of soil eaten and the quantity of concentrates consumed by the ewes. Housing greatly reduces the risk.

N.B. Ministry forecasts are published in the farming and veterinary press.

(d) The grazing is lush. Improved, fertilised and reclaimed pastures are particularly likely to give rise to swayback with single-sward grasses and high Mo and S levels.

(2) *Clinical signs*

(a) *Congenital*

Lambs at or within a few days of birth show varying degrees of ataxia, paresis and inability to stand. Some will be able to suck if permitted and most appear alert and sensible. Some may be born dead, or die within a few hours. The signs are, at best, only suspicious and can easily be confused with the other CNS disturbances of young lambs.

(b) *Delayed*

Lambs a few weeks old, which were normal at birth, developing varying degrees of hind-leg weakness, ataxia (Swayback) and paresis.The signs are more obvious when the lamb is chased about and turns quickly. It looks like a spinal rather than a brain condition and the lambs can suck and graze normally; some will fatten because they learn how to cope with the disability.

(c) *Acute Delayed*

Rapidly developing signs in lambs a few weeks old and dying within a few hours. Uncommon.

(3) *Incidence*

This will depend upon the control measures adopted and the weather but it is common for a swayback-prone farm to have a few years with very few cases, followed by a calamitous 'storm' (50%). Fortunately, the advent of housing and safe copper supplementation has reduced these incidents.

(4) *Pathology:* Material for diagnosis:

(a) Formalinised brains and brain stems.

(b) At least 10 heparinised blood samples (green tubes) from pregnant ewes that have not recently had supplementary copper.

Concentrations below 9µl/litre or 0.07 mg/100ml suggest a copper problem and supplementation is required.

(c) Liver copper concentrations-below 235 µmol or 15mg/kg D.M.

(d) Herbage analysis: Cu – below 5 ppm D.M.

Mo – above 1 ppm D.M.

S -above 0.20% D.M.

Treatment

Because swayback can be a progressive condition, it is worth treating those young lambs which are not too severely affected with a single dose of copper (e.g. 0.5ml i/m of Copavet Injection, C-Vet Ltd.) in an attempt to stop the condition getting worse.

Control

(1) *During an outbreak:*

All the remaining pregnant ewe should be dosed with copper, together with those healthy lambs already born out of ewes not previously dosed, in order to prevent delayed sway-back.

(2) *Next year:*

Consider housing the ewes during the last half of pregnancy, thus removing them from the source of the problem.

If in doubt, dose all ewes in early pregnancy with copper but also then remove other known sources of copper such as copperised licks/minerals and proprietary cattle and pig concentrates.

If there is a problem of ill-thrift, poor quality fleece and multiple fractures in lambs due to copper deficiency, then the lambs also require dosing, but not before other causes have been eliminated and copper deficiency established.

A variety of preparations is available which vary in convenience of use and packaging and in their formulation, which determines the speed of absorption, irritancy and toxicity; you need to pick and choose quite carefully to find the most suitable product for the occasion and the farm.

Injectable preparations

The dose for ewes is 2ml costing approximately 25p.

(1) Quick release (e.g. Cujec, Coopers Pitman-Moore, s/c, and Cuvine , Rycovet Ltd, i/m). Water soluble, rapidly absorbed and therefore potentially more toxic.

(2) Slow release (e.g. Copavet, C-Vet Ltd) Suspension, more slowly absorbed and therefore likely to be safer but more irritant.

Oral preparation

The safest and arguably the most reliable preparations are in the form of capsules containing copper oxide needles (e.g. Copporal, Beecham Animal Health; 4g for ewes costing approx. 35p and 2g for lambs, costing 20p) and delivered by a plastic gun. Ewes are dosed once in mid-pregnancy and lambs as required when they are over 5 weeks old.

Short acting drenches are often used, but they require repeat dosing and risk toxicity. Copacobal Oral Drench (C-Vet Ltd.) contains copper sulphate and cobalt chloride and to prevent swayback, it is given in mid-pregnancy and repeated one month later, costing approximately 5p per dose (10 ml of the diluted preparation). Copper sulphate on its own (1.0g in 30 ml water) is still used prophylactically by farmers, but it is a risky material to have about on sheep farms.

To avoid TOXICITY, either within hours of injection or weeks after dosing:

(1) Make sure copper is necessary.

(2) Reduce dose of injection in small sheep.

(3) Remove any other obvious source of copper, particularly if housed and fed concentrates.

(4) Treat ewes with care, and follow makers' recommendations.

There is evidence that individuals and breeds vary in susceptibility to copper deficiency, e.g. Scottish Blackface and Swaledales are more prone, and a change in breed might be considered, or an alteration in the lambing date, or special precautions for selected breeds, or cull those ewes that produce swayback lambs. Note that high sulphate and molybdenum (Mo) levels in the diet are known to decrease copper 'availability', hence the term 'conditioned' copper deficiency, and hence also the use of ammonium molybdate and sodium sulphate in controlling chronic copper toxicity.

BORDER DISEASE (BD) AND HYPOMYELOGENESIS CONGENITA (HC) 'HAIRY SHAKERS'

This is a congenital disease, first reported from the English-Welsh border counties but since recognised throughout the world. It is caused by infection with a pestivirus (BDV) serologically closely related to Bovine Virus Diarrhoea Virus (BVDV). Antigenic differences can be recognised between BDV and BVDV, but sheep isolates will infect cattle and vice versa. Serological differences between two isolates of BDV have been recognised and sheep which are immune to one isolate are susceptible to the other.

Clinical Picture

BDV infection produces a number of clinical signs, though they do not all occur in every flock. One or more of the following pictures may be seen:

(1) A number of lambs showing a typical long hairy coat, some of which are also ataxic with fine rhythmic tonic/clonic contractions of skeletal muscles. These signs are usually evident at birth, although in the naturally long-woolled breeds, the abnormal birth coat is not obvious. The incidence of BD and HC lambs is variable but 'storms' are reported. Gimmers produce the highest percentage of BD and HC lambs, indicating progressive immunity.

(2) Many affected lambs survive for a time, but their growth rate is poor and they appear stunted with domed heads and lag behind the rest of the flock. In addition, persistently infected lambs occur, many of which do not show the early signs, but some show chronic unthriftiness and scouring. Some survive to breeding age, and though their fertility is reduced, they can produce infected lambs in successive pregnancies. Persistently infected rams can transmit virus in semen.

(3) A high prevalence of barren ewes, abortions, or even of just weak lambs. This means that the disease may show as an abortion and infertility problem rather than as a disease of young lambs.

Pathogenesis

Infection of healthy non-pregnant sheep produces no obvious clinical signs and gives rise to the production of neutralising antibodies and an immune sheep. It is 'antibody positive, virus negative'.

Infection of pregnant ewes leads to a similar course of events in the ewe, but virus crosses the placenta and leads to the various clinical pictures, depending on virus strain and breed of sheep, but most importantly, on the stage of gestation. If infection occurs after about 90 days, the foetus mounts an immunological response and destroys the virus. Most will be normal at birth and will be 'antibody positive, virus negative', like the dam.

Infection prior to 60 days, at a time when the foetus has no ability to mount an immunological response, will result in foetal death in a high proportion of cases, leading to resorption and barren ewes or mummification and abortion. Virus strains vary in virulence and these early infections may allow some infected foetuses to survive with virus in virtually every organ. Infection of CNS leads to myelin deficiency and 'shaker' lambs and of hair follicles leads to'hairy' lambs. Weak or even apparently healthy infected lambs may be produced. All these lambs will be immunologically tolerant to BDV and 'antibody negative, virus positive' at birth, and although they will acquire antibody in the colostrum, this will wane and they will be 'virus positive', probably for life. These lambs are persistent carriers.

If infection occurs between 60 and 90 days, when the foetus is becoming immunologically competent, either of the above responses may occur and either clinical outcome.

Epidemiology

Most flocks become infected by the purchase of persistently infected lambs as breeding replacements. It has been suggested that, rarely, infection may be introduced by pestiviruses from other species such as cattle, goats or deer, or even by a contaminated live vaccine.

Diagnosis

The following indicates the tissues needed for laboratory confirmation of clinical diagnosis.

(1) 'Hairy-shaker', weak, scouring lambs or suspect persistently infected sheep. Clotted blood (red tube) from live lambs for virus isolation and serology. In dead animals, virus can be detected by immunofluorescence and virus isolation from fresh tissues, e.g. kidney, spleen, thyroid. Heart blood may be used for serology. Brain and spinal cord in calcium formol-saline for histology.

(2) Aborting or barren ewes. Clotted blood for virology and serology. Placenta for virus isola tion.

Treatment and Control

There is no treatment and there are dangers in attempting to support weak or hairy shaker lambs which will be excreting virus.

Ideally, a closed flock should be maintained or replacements obtained from a flock which is serologically negative (future ingredient of ADAS Health Scheme?). Maintaining replacements as a separate flock from tupping to lambing will enable monitoring of lambing to be done.

In a flock which has recently had BD for the first time, the sheep suspected of introducing the infection may be identified as 'antibody negative, virus positive' from blood samples. They and their lambs should be culled before the next tupping season.

In an endemically infected flock, all breeding ewes should be deliberately exposed to infection 2 to 3 months before tupping by housing in close contact with persistently infected sheep for 3 to 4 weeks.

It seems likely that vaccines will become available for BD and BVD.

Further reading
Nettleton, P (1988). 'Update- Border Disease' *In Practice*, Vol. 10, 76–8.

DAFT LAMB DISEASE - CONGENITAL CEREBELLAR CORTICAL ATROPHY

A non-febrile disease of the CNS of newborn lambs characterised by faulty cerebellar development and function. It is probably hereditary and is a particular problem in Border Leicesters. It may also be an expression of a maternal infection during early pregnancy (cf. Border Disease).

Distinctive Features

(1) Usually seen at birth, or develops within the first few days of life.

(2) Mentally stupid (daft). Rarely still with aimless wandering.

(3) Head nodding and swaying, sometimes with opisthotonus and the head arched over the back.

(4) Histology - degeneration of Purkinge and Golgi Cells in cerebellum. The myelin is normal and there are normal copper concentrations in the blood and liver.

(5) Incidence is usually low, but it could justify changing the ram and not breeding again from the dams of affected lambs.

CEREBRO-CORTICAL NECROSIS (CCN)

(Polioencephalomalacia, 'brain rot')

This is an acute exciting central nervous disease, mainly affecting lambs 2 to 6 months old (not under 2 months, as it requires a functional rumen), but it does occur occasionally in adults. It usually occurs sporadically and 'out of the blue' but there are occasional outbreaks affecting a small number of sheep, and lasting a few weeks following a history of change in food or worm drenching. It is associated with a deficiency of thiamine probably induced by the microbial (by e.g. *Cl.sporogenes* and *Bacillus thiaminolyticus*) production of thiaminase in the rumen, causing an initial cerebral oedema followed by 'pressure necrosis'.

Clinical signs

After a short period (few hours) of aloofness, dullness and wandering (even circling!), the sheep becomes increasingly excitable (over another few hours even up to 2 days) developing tremors, staggering, recumbency, opisthotonus and galloping movements. It is usually bilaterally blind and often scouring. It may just be found dead; yet another cause of 'sudden death'. The age of the sheep, the duration and the convulsive nature of the disease may help to differentiate it from such conditions as pulpy kidney, listeriosis, gid, pregnancy toxaemia and hypomagnesaemia, but it requires some confidence to avoid a blunderbuss approach at the first visit!

Diagnosis

(1) Clinical signs and response to thiamine treatment.

(2) PME

 (a) bilateral discoloration of cortical gyri and bright white fluorescence under Wood's lamp of sliced cortex.

 (b) histology.

 (c) rumen contents for estimation of thiaminase activity.

(3) Faeces for increased thiaminase activity, and blood samples for increased pyruvate and decreased transketolase activity can give supportive information, but they need special sampling procedures so contact the VI Centre first.

Treatment

200 – 300mg thiamine, e.g. 2–3ml Vitamin B1 (Bimeda UK Ltd.) or 5ml Parentrovite (Beecham Animal Health) i/v (slowly) and i/m, repeat i/m daily for a few days. If the case has been 'caught early' i.e. before much irreversible necrosis, one expects some improvement within hours (not minutes), i.e. the sheep will be quieter and fewer convulsions, and often there is complete recovery within days, although vision often takes longer to return.

Control

It is reasonable to look at the diet and perhaps suggest changing it e.g. remove from that field or take off that concentrate or lick (e.g. molasses) but it is only making a shaky guess. There is some evidence that the contacts may appear not to be thriving and show signs of scouring, so have a look at them too. They might be injected with 500mg thiamine and perhaps given oral B1 and antibiotics, and the roughage increased, but the incidence does not usually justify such intervention.

Ticks
Tick-borne fever
Tick-bite pyaemia
Louping-ill ('trembling')

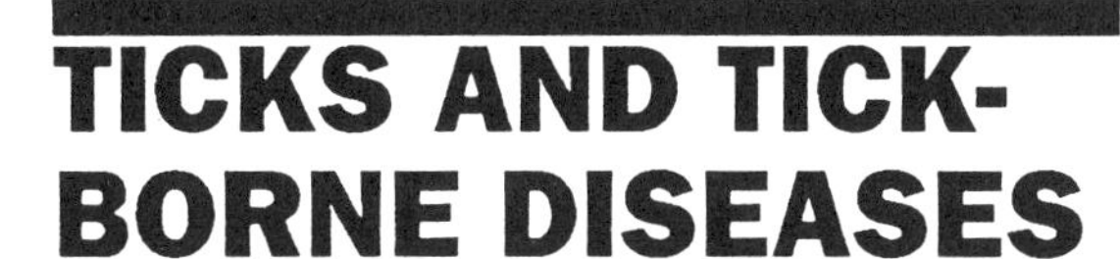

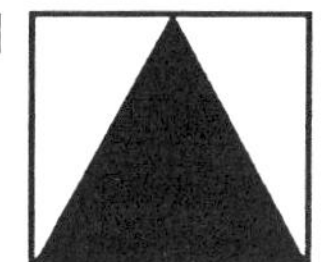

TICKS

The only tick of importance on sheep is *Ixodes ricinus*, the so-called sheep tick, though it is not host-specific. It has a 3 host lifecycle in which less than 3 weeks of the 3 year cycle is spent on the host. Larvae and nymphs can develop successfully on birds and small wild animals, but the adult female needs a large animal host (sheep, cattle, deer) in order to produce eggs. Since 98% of the lifecycle is spent off a host, the success of the tick is very dependent on the external environment.

Geographical distribution

The ticks are dependent on suitable habitats for the stages off the host, which require 100% humidity. The are found, therefore, on rough hill grazing, in Scotland, the Pennines, Lake District, Wales, Devon and Cornwall and a few other small areas. These areas have an annual rainfall of over 100cm (40ins). The vegetation is bracken, heather, rushes and coarse grasses and the number of ticks increase with the thickness of the vegetation matt. Pasture improvement, involving drainage and re-seeding, renders conditions unsuitable for ticks.

Seasonal distribution

In most areas, there is a tick rise in spring and another in autumn, but the precise timing varies from year to year, particularly the time of appearance of the major population in spring. This is always close to lambing, but may occur when lambs are plentiful or sparse, which will influence disease occurrence.

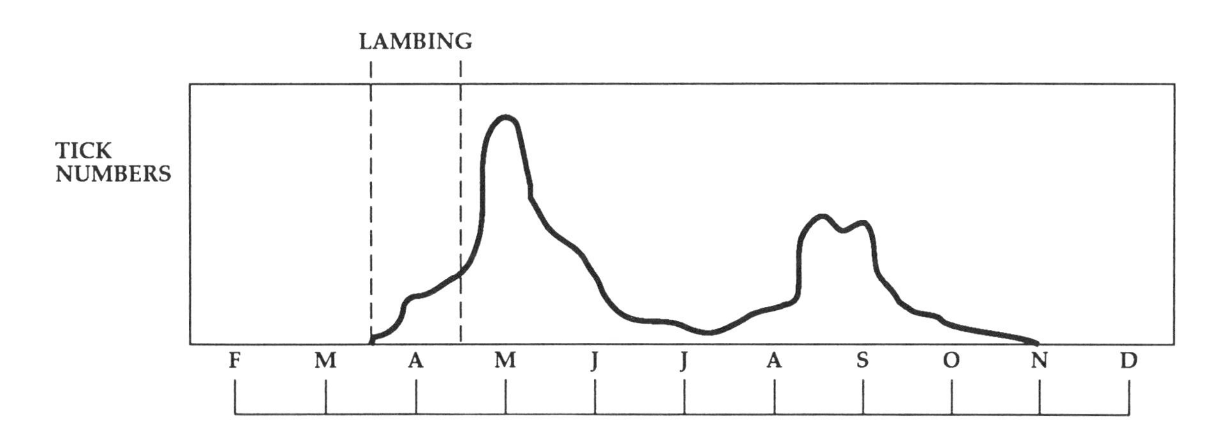

Small numbers of *I.ricinus* can be found on sheep from April to October apart from the peaks, and in a few area (Northumberland and south-east Scotland) there is no autumn rise. Spring rise and autumn rise ticks are different populations.

Flock distribution

The number of ticks found throughout the season on sheep increases with the age (or size) of the sheep. In one count on a heavily infected farm, ewes had 400 adult females, hogs 300 and lambs 50, together with about 5 times as many nymphs as adults, and 1,000 times more larvae than adults.

Sheep distribution

Ticks attach initially to the ears, nose, lips and feet and they migrate to become attached to the hairy parts with only very small numbers in the woolly areas. Adults migrate further than nymphs and larvae hardly migrate at all.

Importance

Ticks are responsible for irritation and a certain amount of blood loss, particularly in young lambs (tick worry) and for the transmission of tick-borne fever, tick-bite pyaemia and louping-ill. The tick-transmitted diseases are more important than tick-worry because heavy infections are uncommon and the blood loss is over a period of some weeks, which allows for compensation.

Control

Tick control is often effected by improvement in grazing associated with increases in stocking rate. It can be done by pasture improvement and by chemical treatment of sheep.

(1) *Pasture Improvement*

Many hill farms are draining and re-seeding the relatively low pastures bordering on the high hills in order to improve lambing percentage and live-weight gains in the lambs. This has a dramatic effect on tick populations which rapidly disappear. If some grazing is improved and is used for ewes late in pregnancy and early in lactation, a waning of immunity to tick-borne disease (especially louping-ill) may result followed by disease when the sheep are later turned on to the tick-infested hill grazings. A similar problem may occur with sheep which are away-wintered on lowland pastures. Heather burning every 5–7 years reduces tick populations.

(2) *Chemical treatment of sheep*

There is a variety of compounds available as dips, 'pour-ons' and 'spot-ons'. One group comprise organo-phosphorus (OP) compounds (e.g. chlorpyrifos, Killtick, Youngs Animal Health) which are diluted and used as a dip. OP compounds, especially the concentrate, are toxic to man and protective clothing must be worn during the dipping procedure. Chlorpyrifos has been used to kill ticks on habitats by spraying in spring- costs are about £15/ha.

Most tick dips are suitable for the control of blowfly, lice and keds and some are approved by MAFF for sheep scab control. Most preparations give protection for 4 weeks in ewes, though some claim to give partial protection for up to 8 weeks. Lambs are protected for only 2–3 weeks.

Ewes are dipped to reduce the pasture infestation in successive years and lambs are protected to try and reduce the number of ticks which they pick up. It is recommended that all ewes should be dipped either before lambing at the end of March or beginning of April or preferably after lambing before going to the fell. All lambs should be dipped or rubbed with salve before going to the fell. Lambs may be dipped from 4 days old, preferably by hand in a 45 gallon drum. Mis-mothering is prevented by:

(a) Allowing an hour after gathering and before dipping.

(b) Drawing off batches of about 20 ewes with their lambs.

(c) Allowing lambs to drain and mother-up before putting a fresh batch through the dip.

Sheep should be re-dipped in autumn.

The other main group comprises synthetic pyrethroids and are applied as a 'pour-on' or 'spot-on'. An example of a 'pour-on' preparation is 2.5% cypermethrin (e.g. Parasol, Ciba-Geigy; Cypor, Youngs Animals Health Ltd) which is applied to the sheep with a special gun in a line from the crown of the head to the top of the rump, but avoiding the tail to prevent mis-mothering. The drug is not active systemically but spreads over the skin surface in the sebum. It will control ticks for up to 12 weeks and is particularly useful in lambs (dose 5–10 ml costing 10–20p) with protection for 3–4 weeks.

An example of a 'spot-on' preparation is deltamethrin (e.g. Spot-on, Coopers Pitman-Moore) which is applied to the skin between the shoulder blades. Protection lasts for 4–6 weeks. Operators must wear protective clothing with synthetic pyrethroids.

TICK-BORNE FEVER (TBF)

This is caused by a rickettsia, *Cytoecetes phagocytophila.* A similar organism of close antigenic identity is found in cattle. The organism is transmitted by the nymph and adult of *I.ricinus* and virtually every tick is infected.

The rickettsia invades the circulating neutrophils and monocytes and results in their destruction, thus causing a neutropenia. It is this feature, combined with a pyrexia, which gives rise to clinical signs and predisposes the sheep to tick pyaemia and increases the severity of louping-ill.

Clinical picture

Since most ticks are infected, lambs in a tick area become infected very early in life. The clinical signs are mild and are usually not noticed - the lambs may be listless, fail to suck and have a temperature rise (up to 41°C) for a few days. There is some evidence that some strains are more pathogenic than others. Organisms can be found by Giemsa stain of a thin blood film. Immunity then develops, is probably short-lived but is reinforced throughout life producing 'acclimatised' sheep. There are no antibodies to TBF in the colostrum, so lambs become infected as soon as they encounter ticks. More severe signs are seen in adult sheep brought from a tick-free area. The high temperature which follows exposure to ticks may result in abortion in pregnant ewes (unusual because the time of year is usually wrong) and temporary infertility (for about 3 months) in rams. This is of considerable importance since rams are usually purchased at September/October sales and are infertile just at the time that they are turned out with the ewes.

Control

The organism is susceptible to sulphonamides and broad spectrum antibiotics, but it is more important to obtain satisfactory immunity in lambs and to produce acclimatised sheep. Do not move non-immune rams or pregnant ewes into a tick area, at least during the breeding season.

TICK-BITE PYAEMIA

This is a generalised infection with *Staphylococcus aureus*, a normal skin commencal, of lambs of 2 to 16 weeks old associated with tick bites and usually predisposed by tick-borne fever. Neutropenic lambs have been shown to be highly susceptible to staphylococcal septicaemia. The disease is either a septicaemia resulting in death or the bacteria localise in many organs, producing abscesses in joints, CNS, liver, lungs, etc. Lambs are rarely infected before two weeks of age, probably because the neutropenia from tick-borne fever is not evident before this time, and also because titres of staphylococcal antibodies derived from the colostrum wane at about two weeks.

Clinical signs

These vary with the site of the abscesses and include lameness with painful enlarged joints, paralysis of the hind legs due to abscess in the spinal cord, signs of meningitis or unthriftiness due to abscesses in liver, lungs, kidneys etc.

The septicaemic form shows in sudden deaths. The disease occurs wherever *I.ricinus* is found and is of great economic importance. It has been shown that half the lamb losses on a tick farm can be due to pyaemia and that virtually all the lameness in lambs is associated with tick-bite pyaemia.

Treatment

Antibiotics (e.g. penicillin) are effective against the organism and if lambs are treated early, the clinical signs may regress and the lambs recover. Lambs with spinal abscesses or with multiple abscesses in liver and lungs are unlikely to recover despite treatment, and it has been suggested that penicillin only hastens the recovery of lambs which were likely to recover spontaneously.

Control

(1) Tick control and control of tick-borne fever. Synthetic pyrethroids applied to 7 day old lambs before putting on tick habitats will delay infection until they are 4 weeks old, and disease is then much less severe.

(2) Long-acting penicillin or tetracycline have been employed prophylactically just prior to exposure to ticks, when the lambs are sent with the ewes to the fell, but these only last for a few days and are not likely to influence disease significantly.

(3) Staphylococcal toxoid. Two doses before exposure might be useful, but lambs do not respond well before six weeks of age. By vaccinating the ewe during pregnancy, it has been possible to induce passive immunity in the lamb for only two weeks. Thus this method is of little practical value.

LOUPING-ILL ('Trembling')

This is a virus disease which affects sheep and many other hosts, including cattle, deer, man and red grouse. Typically, there is an initial viraemia about 2 to 6 days after the tick bite, during which there is a febrile reaction (42°C). The majority of acclimatised sheep show few clinical signs and even susceptible sheep will usually recover rapidly. In some sheep, however, the virus invades the CNS and severe clinical signs and death follow. There is evidence that a primary TBF infection at the same time increases the likelihood of invasion. The virus is transmitted stage to stage by *I.ricinus* and only about 1 in 1000 ticks is infected. Some tick areas have no louping-ill virus present at all.

Clinical signs

Disease is seen in all ages of sheep from as early as 2 days old (? prenatal infection) to aged ewes. Lambs are dependent on colostral immunity for protection, which is strongest when immune ewes are exposed to re-infection a few weeks before lambing. Changes in grazing practice may prevent this natural boost to the immunity of the ewes and many lambs may then become clinically affected. Lambs may be found dead, but the typical signs are those associated with CNS involvement and are variable in nature. They include resting the head on the ground, head-pressing, and abnormal jerky gait ('leaping'), staggering, circling and paralysis. Fine tremors of the facial muscles and ears, nystagmus and twitching or nibbling of the lips may be seen. The disease progresses within 1 to 4 days to coma and death, often assisted by predators.

Usually only a small proportion of the flock is affected, but outbreaks may be explosive with a high mortality. Animals which have recovered from the viraemia have a solid life-long immunity, and specific antibody can be detected in their blood.

Diagnosis in a severe outbreak is usually made on clinical grounds but CCN, listeriosis, swayback, gid or abscesses must be considered. There is a typical histology of the brain and virus can be recovered at the V I Centre by mouse inoculation. There is a serological test for antibody.

Treatment and control

Treatment is not effective but careful nursing indoors may save some cases.

The aim of control is to ensure that ewes are immune and that lambs are protected passively. There is an inactivated vaccine available (Louping-ill vaccine, BP (Vet), Coopers Pitman-Moore) which costs about £1.50/dose and is a white oily emulsion. Warming of the vaccine at body temperature facilitates injection. The recommended procedure for ewes is that 1 ml should be injected subcutaneously between tupping and mid-pregnancy and not later than a month before lambing with a boost every other year before lambing. It may be necessary to protect ewe-lamb replacements before the autumn tick rise.

A summary of possible control methods for ticks and the diseases they transmit is:

(1) Dip ewes around lambing and on 2 occasions later in the summer to reduce tick populations.

(2) Dip or apply pour-on or spot-on preparations to lambs before returning to tick areas.

(3) Penicillin or tetracycline LA to lambs before returning to tick areas.

(4) Special care over introduction of new rams and ewes.

(5) Vaccinate ewes against louping-ill every other year and lambs before the autumn rise.

(6) Heather burning of areas on the fells on a 7 year rotation.

Further reading

Reid, H (1987). 'Controlling tick-borne diseases of sheep in Britain', *In Practice*, Vol. 9, 189–91

Coccidiosis
Parasitic-gastro-enteritis (PGE)
Anthelmintics
Cobalt deficiency
Nephrosis

THIN SCOURING LAMBS

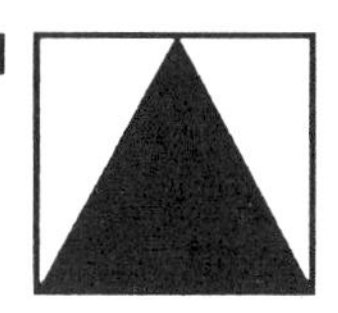

A considerable number of causes of scouring lambs over a month old have been described, and loss of condition always accompanies chronic diarrhoea. Possible causes are salmonellosis, Campylobacter infection, ingestion of fertiliser from recently treated pastures and Border Disease, but the most important, common causes are coccidiosis and parasitic gastroenteritis. Mineral deficiencies, particularly of cobalt, lead to unthriftiness without scouring unless parasites are present also.

COCCIDIOSIS

The incidence of coccidiosis, as recorded by VIC figures, has increased steadily over the last 10–15 years and is recognised as a considerable hazard of intensively reared lambs. About a dozen species of *Eimeria* have been described which are specific to sheep, and their pathogenicity differ considerably. Many of them produce few if any clinical signs, whereas two species (*E. ovinoidalis* and *E. crandallis*) may cause severe disease, characterised by diarrhoea, weight loss and death.

History

The majority of outbreaks, which involve a high proportion of the lambs, occur in animals of 4 to 8 weeks old which have been housed since birth, or grazed on constantly used pasture at very high stocking rates.

Epidemiology

The ewes act as a source of oocysts and sporulation occurs in 2 or 3 days in the bedding. Oocysts remain viable for up to a year.

The peak incidence at 6–8 weeks of age was believed to be due to the fact that one cycle had to take place in the lambs, taking 2–3 weeks, in order to build up a heavy environmental contamination with oocysts. Disease resulted from the multiplication of this second cycle in the intestine before an effective immunity had developed. Recently, however, it has been shown that lambs are not susceptible to coccidial infections early in life and that susceptibility increases up to 4–6 weeks of age. If heavy infections are encountered early in life, clinical signs are not seen (due to passive transfer of immunity?), active immunity is stimulated and the lambs are less likely to show clinical signs of coccidiosis at 4–8 weeks old. After this age, most lambs have encountered infection and develop a strong immunity.

Clinical signs

The first sign is that the farmer may recognise that the lambs have lost 'bloom' and show an 'open' fleece. Some animals may have slight diarrhoea with soiling of the wool below the anus. These signs extend to a considerable number of the flock and weight gains are reduced, followed by weight loss. Severe untreated cases proceed to extensive scouring, dehydration and death. Treated recovered lambs often continue to make poor weight gains due to slow repair of the intestinal lesions.

Diagnosis

This is based on clinical signs and history. Oocyst counts are not reliable since it is possible to see clinical coccidiosis associated with developing sexual stages, before peak oocyst production occurs, and counts of up to 1 million oocysts per g can be seen without clinical signs. It has been stated that it is easier to arrive at a diagnosis of coccidiosis if you don't possess a microscope! Nevertheless, it is often helpful to examine a number of faecal samples (say 10) when counts of over 100,000 oocyst per g in some samples, together with suggestive clinical signs and history, warrant treatment for coccidiosis. In lambs out at grass, *Nematodirus battus* infection should be considered, and concurrent infection with *E. ovinoidalis*, *E. crandallis* and *N. battus* is known to cause a severe disease. It is useful to sporulate and identify the species of Eimeria, but this is a specialist job.

Treatment

(1) Orally with sulphonamides (e.g. an initial dose of 2.5ml/5kg body wt of 33.3% solution of Sulphadimidine followed by half this dose for 2 days).

(2) Parenterally with 1ml/10kg body wt of sulphamethoxpyridazine (Parke-Davis 'Midicel Parenteral') for one or two days.

(3) Orally with 1ml/10kg body wt of amprolium/ethopabate (MSD Agvet 'Amprol-Plus' Solution) daily for 4 or 5 days.

Prevention

On farms on which coccidiosis occurs regularly, strategic treatment with the drugs mentioned for treatment may be given to all lambs at 3 and 6 weeks old.

Drugs may be incorporated into lambs' creep feed from birth, but lambs do not eat much creep feed if the ewes are producing large quantities of milk. A very palatable creep feed containing the coccidiostat, salinomycin was marketed by Hoechst Animal Health (Ovicox), but this was expensive and is no longer available. Decoquinate (Deccox Sheep Premix, RMB Animal Health Ltd) and Monensin (Romensin Premix, Elanco Products Ltd) can be incorporated into creep feed.

PARASITIC GASTRO-ENTERITIS (PGE)

PGE is the most important cause of thin, scouring lambs from as early as 2 months of age up to about a year old. During the first year of life a strong immunity develops which not only means that clinical signs are rarely, if ever, seen but also means that sheep may ingest infective larvae (L_3), but the lifecycle is not completed and egg counts are very low for most of the year. The important exception to this rule is the periparturient rise in faecal egg count in ewes and the frequent observation that adult rams may have high egg counts.

The important worms in Britain are *Ostertagia* species in the abomasum and *Trichostrongylus* and *Nematodirus* species in the small intestine. Explosive outbreaks of *Haemonchus* infection in the abomasum are seen, particularly in Southern England in July and August.

Clinical signs

Nematodirus battus causes severe scouring, loss of bloom, dehydration, loss in condition and death in lambs in May and June. Ewes are not affected and immunity develops rapidly in the lambs.

Ostertagia, Trichostrongylus and *Nematodirus filicollis* contribute in different proportions to PGE during the rest of the year, usually commencing in July and continuing in the late winter with chronic scouring and unthriftiness. Subclinical parasitism characterised by reduced weight gains without significant scouring is probably of even greater economic importance than the more obvious clinical signs.

Haemonchus, which differs from the other worms in being an active blood sucker, leads to anaemia, loss in condition and death, without scouring.

Life cycles and epidemiology

N. battus has a very long lifecycle with, typically, only one cycle in 12 months. Eggs, which can be distinguished from those of other worms, develop slowly and overwinter as a third stage larva within the egg. After being exposed to a low temperature over the winter, the L_3 hatch when the temperature rises to above 10°C, thus resulting in a heavy pasture infestation over a short period in the spring. The MAFF issue a nematodiriasis forecast every spring based on soil temperatures, which allow the forecasting of the time of the mass hatch. If this is early (e.g. February/March), most spring-born lambs will not ingest many L_3, since they will have died off before the lambs are consuming much grass. If, however, there is a late winter and the mass hatch does not occur until May, severe disease is likely since the older lambs will be eating a considerable quantity of grass. The cycle is essentially a lamb-to-lamb annual infection.

With *Ostertagia* and *Trichostrongylus*, the eggs, which are indistinguishable from each other (or from *Haemonchus*) develop to a first stage larva which hatches. The L_3 is the infective stage and the time taken for an egg to develop to L_3 varies with the environmental temperature from as little as 2 weeks to as long as 4 months. Eggs are produced for a few weeks by ewes of all ages around lambing time and during lactation by the 'activation' of inhibited L_4 in the mucosa and by lambs which eat L_3 with the pasture. L_3 overwinter on the pasture and die off rapidly during May and June. Pastures which are grazed by sheep every year are contaminated, therefore, by two main methods - by overwintered L_3 and by L_3 which develop from the periparturient egg rise of ewes.

Diagnosis

PGE should be suspected from the clinical signs, the history of a high proportion of the lambs being involved, and can usually be confirmed by faecal egg counts on a number of affected lambs. Egg counts are usually over 1000 eggs per g of faeces though, with *N. battus* in particular, severe scouring can occur just before the worms become mature and produce eggs. *Haemonchus* infections produce high egg counts of 5–10 000 epg. Worm counts on dead or killed lambs in the abomasum and first 10 metres of small intestine will usually yield counts of 50 000 or more, but many may be immature.

Control

It is very important that an effective control programme is produced for lowland intensive sheep flocks, so that not only obvious clinical signs are prevented but the reduced weight gains associated with subclinical infections are avoided. An effective parasite control scheme results in lambs being sent for slaughter much more rapidly, usually resulting in improved economic performance and simplifying management.

Pastures may be categorised as 'clean' or 'dirty', depending on whether they had sheep on in the previous year. The control methods differ in the two systems.

Clean grazing

Clean grazing systems have been pioneered by the East of Scotland College of Agriculture, and providing they are rigidly adhered to, and incorporate a 3 year rotation of cattle, sheep and conservation, considerably increased weight gains are produced with very low pasture L_3. Since the only source of infection is the periparturient rise in ewe faecal egg count, the only anthelmintic treatment which is needed is around lambing time, though, in housed sheep, this dose can be given any time after housing provided the drug chosen is effective against inhibited L_4. Recently, there have been breakdowns of clean grazing systems based on 2 year rotations of cattle-sheep since *N. battus* has become adapted to cattle, and *Cooperia oncophora* to sheep. Pasture contamination is not then broken in the year in which the 'unnatural' host is grazing.

Dirty grazing

Unfortunately, many farms cannot operate a clean grazing system since cattle and sheep numbers are not balanced. Anthelmintics can be used to control infection by frequent dosing in the spring, when clinical signs are not present, in order to prevent heavy L_3 infestation on the pasture in July/August.

The ewes are treated to prevent the periparturient rise as previously described, but further treatments must be given after turn-out since the ingestion of overwintered L_3 by a ewe whose immune response is reduced, will result in the completion of the lifecycle and resulting egg contamination of the pasture. Since the prepatent period of the worms is 3 weeks, treatment must be at this interval. Ewes are dosed, therefore, 3 and 6 weeks after turn-out, by which time their immunity is becoming re-established and their egg count falling naturally.

Since the lambs will start to eat significant quantities of grass containing L_3 by the time they are 4 weeks old, they should be treated at 6 weeks (with the last ewe dose) and at 3 week intervals until the overwintered L_3 have undergone considerable mortality, say, until one treatment in June.

Although many farmers believe that gathering ewes and lambs for dosing at 3 and 6 weeks old will result in mis-mothering, this does not occur in practice, especially if the ewes are separated with their lambs in lots of 50 or so.

Treatment

Although we possess a large number of highly effective anthelmintics (see Table), treatment of severely affected lambs often has little effect in improving weight gains or stopping the scouring. This may be due to anthelmintic resistance, but is more often due to the heavy pasture infections which mean that lambs continue to ingest L_3 and/or to only slowly-reversible gastro-intestinal pathology. Lambs should be treated and moved to a clean pasture, such as aftermath, to avoid continued infection.

ANTHELMINTICS

There are now so many effective anthelmintics available against sheep parasites that a selective approach has been used in this book. The anthelmintics are divided into the main chemical groupings, since this knowledge is of value for the annual rotation of drugs to reduce the development of anthelmintic resistance and examples of each are given. The mention of a particular example does not imply that we have evidence that this proprietary preparation is more effective than others of the same group. An attempt has been made to produce a more extensive list of drugs in the Table (page 86). Comments based on published data on relative efficacy will be found in the text dealing with the different parasitic diseases.

Anthelmintics for nematode infections

(1) *Benzimadazoles and probenzimidazoles (which are metabolised to benzimidazoles)*

These are the most widely used drugs for the treatment and control of parasitic gastroenteritis, accounting for about 80% of the market in Britain. The first member, thiabendazole (still available as Thibenzole), was introduced in 1961 and is the parent drug from which the large number of benzimidazoles have been derived.

All benzimidazoles (except triclabendazole – see Fluke) are effective against all stages of the normal lifecycle of the worms which cause parasitic gastroenteritis (PGE) (e.g. Oxibendazole), some are also effective against lung worms (e.g. Mebendazole); and some are effective against inhibited 4th stage larvae, involved in Type II Ostertagiasis (e.g. Fenbendazole). They cost about 8p a dose for a 25kg lamb, are PML products and have withdrawal periods for meat of 0 (Thiabendazole) to 14 days (Fenbendazole), which may be of importance when lambs are marketed weekly. Some may be used in milking sheep with withdrawal periods of 0 (Thiabendazole) to 3 days (Fenbendazole). Some drugs are not recommended for use in milking sheep (e.g. Mebendazole). They are available in a wide range of formulations including a drench suspension, feed pellets, feed block, powders or intraruminal injections. Oral preparations containing cobalt and selenium also are common. It is probable that slow release preparations will become available commercially since they are now undergoing field trials.

Anthelmintic resistance to one benzimidazole is virtually certain to mean that the worms will be resistant to all benzimidazoles and probenzimidazoles.

(2) *Imidazothiazoles*

The one anthelmintic in this group is levamisole, the l-isomer of tetramisole. Originally marketed as Nilverm, there are now dozens of proprietary formulations. Levamisole is effective against all stages of the lifecycle of worms responsible for PGE, including inhibited larvae and against lungworm infection. The different preparations cost 6–10p a dose for a 25kg lamb and have withdrawal periods of 3 days for meat and 1 day for milk. Levamisole is available as feed granules and as a solution, which may be given orally, by subcutaneous injection or as a 'pour-on'.

(3) *Avermectins*

The one anthelmintic in this group is ivermectin, marketed as Oramec drench for sheep though there is an injectable preparation for cattle and pigs (Ivomec injection, MSD Agvet). It is effective against all stages of worms causing PGE, including inhibited larvae, against lungworm infection (and against nasal botfly). It costs 13p for a 25kg lamb and has a withdrawal period of 14 days for meat and 28 days for milk.

(4) *Tetrahydropyrimidines*

There is no sheep preparation of anthelmintics in this group available in Britain though Morantel and Pyrantel (Pfizer Ltd) available for use in other species are examples.

(5) *Other drugs*

Some drugs, which are mainly used against fluke infections, are also effective against the blood sucking nematode, *H.contortus*. Examples are closantel (Flukiver), and nitroxynil (Trodax). They have been used in worm control programmes against benzimidazole resistant strains in Australasia.

Anthelmintic resistance

The ability of some sheep nematodes to survive treatment with anthelmintics at the normal recommended dose has been reported from many countries, and is particularly important in warm countries in the Southern hemisphere. Resistance occurs when husbandry practices exert a strong selective pressure on the population of worms which allows individuals with resistant genes to increase. Resistance has been described to all the main groups of anthelmintics in Australia and South Africa but, fortunately, is much less common in Britain. Benzimidazole resistance of *H.contortus* has been shown to occur widely in farms in Southern England, necessitating the use of other anthelmintics for its control. Although there are few reports of resistance to benzimidazoles and levamisole in *Ostertagia* and *Trichostrongylus* species in Britain, most studies have indicated that resistance to these worms is very rare and probably, at present, of little importance.

Before deciding that failure to respond to anthelmintics is due to resistance, checks should be made that a correct dose has been given (weigh sheep, calculate a precise dose rather than the range recommended by the manufacturers and check volume delivered by gun) and that heavy reinfection or irreversible pathology are not responsible. A useful on-farm test for resistance is to take faeces for egg counts from 10 lambs before treatment of 5 of them, and resample 7–10 days later. Modern anthelmintics are virtually 100% effective – the 5 untreated lambs allow normal fluctuations to be monitored but are probably not essential. Culture of any eggs remaining after treatment to L_3 allow a species identification to be made. Laboratory tests are available to determine resistance, but the most reliable method is by a controlled test involving experimental infections. If drug resistance is indicated by the on-farm egg count reduction test described above, the company who market the anthelmintic should be informed.

Anthelmintics for fluke infections

There is no published evidence to indicate that fluke (*Fasciola hepatica*) have become resistant to anthelmintics and drugs are selected mainly on their efficacy at normally recommended doses, against different stages of the parasite.

Oxyclozanide and albendazole are effective only against adult flukes, nitroxynil, rafoxanide and closantel are effective against immature fluke of about 6 weeks old and triclabendazole and diamphenethide are effective against all ages of fluke.

Anthelmintics for cestode infections

Adult tape worms of the genus *Moniezia* are extremely common in young lambs and strings of white segments are frequently seen by farmers in the faeces and blamed for any clinical signs which may be found at the same time. There is little evidence that they exert any adverse effect on production. However, many benzimidazoles (e.g. albendazole, oxfendazole), are very effective against *Moniezia*. It should not be forgotten that sheep act as intermediate hosts for several cestodes of the dog and that treatment of dogs should form part of a sheep health programme (see page 35).

Anthelmintics for sheep This list is not exhaustive. It has been prepared from IVS, October 1989 and Compendium of Data Sheets, 1989–90

Chemical name	Trade name	Company (abb)	Dose mg/kg	Cost (p)* 25kg lamb	Formulation	Activity G	I	L	T	F	Withdrawal period (days) Meat	Milk
Benzimidazoles												
Albendazole	Valbazen	Smith K	5	10	Suspension	+	+	+	+	+	10	NU
	Bental	Rycovet	7.5 fluke							(adults)		
Fenbendazole	Panacur	Hoechst	5	9	Suspension powder pellets feedblock	+	+	+	+	-	14	3
Mebendazole	Ovitelmin	Janssen	15	10	Suspension	+	-	+	+	-	7	1
Oxfendazole	Synanthic	Syntex	5	11	Suspension intra ruminal injection	+	+	+	+	-	14	2
	Systamex	Wellcome	5	11	Suspension	+	+	+	+	-	14	2
Oxibendazole	Widespec	Rycovet	10	7	Suspension	+	-	-	-	-	4	3
	Anthelworm	Young	10	7	Suspension	+	-	-	-	-	4	3
Netobimin	Hapadex	Kirkby-Warwick	7.5 (20 fluke, inh.L4)	6	Suspension	+	+	+	+	+ (adults)	5	3
Thiabendazole	Thibenzole	MSD	44	10	Suspension paste (+Co) powder pellets	+	-	+	-	-	0	0
Triclabendazole	Fasinex	Ciba-Geigy	10	5	Suspension	-	-	-	-	+	28	NU
Probenzimadazoles												
Febantel	Bayverm	Bayer	5	9	Suspension pellets	+	+	+	+	-	8	2
Thiophanate	Nemafax	RMB	50	7	Suspension pellets	+	-	+	-	-	7	3
Imidazothiazoles												
Levamisole	Many preparations eg. Cevasol (Ceva) Cyverm (Cyanamid) Duphamisole (Duphar) Levacide (Norbrook) Levadin (Univet) Bionem, Nilverm (Coopers) Ripercol (Janssen)		7.5	7	Solution granules (oral, s/c injection) depending on manufacturer	+	+	+	-	-	3	1
Avermectins												
Ivermectin	Oramec	MSD	0.2	13	Solution	+	+	+	+	-	14	NU
Other drugs (mainly for fascioliasis)												
Closantel	Flukiver	Janssen	10	6	Suspension	-**	-	-	-	+	28	NU
Diamphenethide	Coriban	Coopers	100	18	Suspension	-	-	-	-	+	7	NU
Nitroxynil	Trodax	RMB	10	5	Solution (20%) (s/c injection)	-**	-	-	-	+	30	NU
Oxyclozanide	Zanil	Coopers	15	9	Suspension granules	-	-	-	-	+ (adults)	14	0
Rafoxanide	Flukanide	MSD	7.5	4	Suspension injection	-	-	-	-	+	28	NU

There are also a number of preparations which are a combination of drugs active against nematodes and fluke, eg.
Duospec (Rycovet), oxibendazole/oxyclozanide
Flukombin (Bayer)
Vermadex (RMB), thiophanate/brotianide
Nilzan (Coopers), levamisole/oxyclozanide
Ranizole (MSD), thiabendazole/rafoxanide.

G - Gastro-intestinal nematodes
I - inhibited L_4
L - lungworm
T - tapeworm
F - fluke

* This is given for comparative purposes. All these products are PML and the price is that given in the Index of Veterinary Specialities, October 1989.
** Active against *Haemonchus* and other blood sucking worms.

NU – not to be used for sheep producing milk for human consumption.

COBALT DEFICIENCY

Cobalt deficiency is the cause of 'pine' or 'ill-thrift' in lambs. The incidence is highest in areas where soils are derived from acid igneous rocks and where there are coarse, sandy soils. In Scotland, cobalt deficiency is widely distributed but in England, the localities most likely to be deficient are in the limestone areas of the Pennines, the Old Red Sandstone areas of Hereford, Shropshire and Worcester, Dartmoor and the Greensands at the edge of the chalk in south-east England. As well as these areas where cobalt deficiency is endemic, other areas have become cobalt deficient as a result of farming practices, such as liming and reseeding which have improved pastures and in so doing, lowered the available cobalt. A constant intake of cobalt is needed to allow rumen organisms to produce vitamin B12, and the disease caused by cobalt deficiency is thus an induced vitamin B12 deficiency.

Clinical signs

The typical disease is characterised by loss of appetite, reduced weight gains proceeding to weight loss and extreme emaciation. Lambs have a dry coat and a tight skin. In the terminal stages, there is severe anaemia and lachrymation. Subclinically, a marginal deficiency of cobalt may be of considerable economic importance since typical signs may not be present but weight gains may be reduced. Parasitic gastro-enteritis is often also present and its clinical effects are more serious, and copper deficiency may be a complicating factor causing reduced growth rate in hill areas where pasture improvement has been carried out. However, farmers tend to suspect deficiency states with little evidence so care should be taken over diagnosis.

The adult ewe may show signs of deficiency in late pregnancy due to fatty liver leading to perinatal mortality.

Diagnosis

(1) History of farm and geographical area.

(2) Clinical findings.

(3) Response to treatment. This is often very marked after cobalt administration, but it should be noted that lambs with reduced appetite due to other causes may also show a response to dosing with cobalt.

(4) Laboratory confirmation:

In the animal (sample at least 10 animals)

(a) Serum vitamin B12 concentration

Adequate: over 400 ng/l (300 pmol/l)

Marginal: 200–400 ng/l (150–300 pmol/l)

Deficient: less than 200 ng/l (150 pmol/l)

Different assay systems produce somewhat different results and the laboratory may indicate slightly different values from these for deficiency.

(b) Liver vitamin B12 concentration.

Deficient: less than 1 μg/g dry tissue

Serum and liver vitamin B12 concentrations are insensitive indicators of deficiency but good indices of excess. The uncertainties of interpretation of serum and liver vitamin B12 concentrations led to tests designed to measure the functional significance of vitamin B12.

(c) Urinary metabolites-methyl malonic acid (MMA) and formiminoglutamic acid (FIGLU).

Vitamin B12 deficiency causes a depression in propionate metabolism and it, and MMA, a product of propionate metabolism, builds up and MMA is excreted in the urine.

FIGLU is an intermediary product of histidine catabolism, and its own catabolism requires the presence of vitamin B12. It, like MMA, therefore accumulates in the urine of deficient lambs.

FIGLU is not a reliable indicator of subclinical deficiency, however, since pronounced clinical signs including loss of weight are necessary for it to accumulate whereas MMA starts to accumulate somewhat earlier. It is now possible to detect the elevation of MMA in the blood, rising rapidly above normal (5µmol/l) when vitamin B12 falls below 300 ng/l (Urine can often be obtained in sheep by partial suffocation!)

In the food:

(a) Herbage deficiency is likely to follow when below 0.11 mg Co/kg DM, since this is the dietary requirement.

(b) Soil – deficiency when below 0.3 mg Co/kg DM.

Treatment and prevention

There is no placental transfer of B12 and only low concentrations in milk; lambs require colostrum for their first supply.

(1) *Cobalt pellets* (often called 'bullets')

The most effective treatment is to give each lamb, at about 8 weeks of age (not before, because they are too small to dose, and the rumen is not fully developed) a cobalt pellet (e.g. Permaco S, Coopers Pitman-Moore). This should be effective for at least a year, but it costs approximately 60p per pellet, and for fattening lambs it may not be worth it, though it would be for ewe lambs which are to be kept for breeding.

(2) *Oral dosing with cobalt*

A drench can be made by dissolving 100g of cobalt sulphate in 2 litres of water to provide a stock solution. 250ml of this stock solution is then diluted in 5 litres of water; give young lambs 10ml (less than 0.5p), older lambs 15ml and adult ewes (where necessary) 30ml. This will need to be repeated every 3 weeks.

C-Vet Ltd produce a preparation 'Copacobal', containing copper and cobalt, which costs approximately 5p per dose and only 2 doses are advised (at 8 weeks and again in the autumn), but this seems to be an unusually long interval to be really effective.

Several anthelmintics are available combined with cobalt (and selenium), so regular anthelmintic dosing also helps to prevent Co deficiency. Provided the deficiency is not severe, this is an easy way of dealing with worms and cobalt deficiency.

(3) *Cobalt supplementation in mineral mixture or water*

It is unlikely that lambs will be on concentrates but if so, the mineral mixture should contain sufficient cobalt to raise the whole feed to 0.11mg Co/kg DM. Cobalt supplementation of water supply is suitable only for sheep receiving piped water. Cobalt sulphate is dissolved and kept in a concentrated solution in a metering device plumbed into the water supply, in such a way as to deliver a known, steady amount of cobalt. The method is cheap, after initial installation of equipment, and animals need the minimum of handling.

(4) *Injection of vitamin B12*

This will deal rapidly with an immediate problem, but cost and the need for injections every 3 weeks precludes this as a preventive measure. There are several preparations and the dose for sheep is about 500µg, costing about 10p.

(5) *Application of cobalt sulphate to grazing land*

Cobalt sulphate may be applied as a spray or as a granular top-dressing at 2.0 kg per hectare. Dressing need only be repeated every 3 years (or 6 years if the deficiency is only marginal) and only one-third of the grazing need be treated (at 6 kg/ha), since the sheep graze the treated strip selectively. The pasture should not be treated soon after liming. The cost of cobalt sulphate preparations varies markedly but will be in the region of 15p per lamb.

Further reading
Mitchell, G and Linklater, K (1983). 'Differential diagnosis of scouring in lambs', *In Practice*, Vol. 5, 4–12.
MAFF. *Clean grazing systems for sheep*, Booklet Number 2324.
Taylor, M A and Hunt, K R (1989). 'Anthelmintic drug resistance in the UK', *Veterinary Record*, Vol. 125, 143–47.

NEPHROSIS

Although it has been recognised that renal damage leading to acute renal failure in lambs of 8–16 weeks old is occasionally seen in association with outbreaks of *Nematodirus battus* infection, a number of centres have recently reported nephrosis in much younger lambs.

Clinical signs

Lambs of any age over 7 days up to about 10 weeks old may be affected. The young ones, up to about 4 weeks old, show very few signs other than being inexplicably dull and unable to suck; they rapidly become comatose and die within a few days. Older lambs are often unthrifty and are scouring, which leads one to suspect parasitic gastro-enteritis and the farmer to treat with anticoccidials and/or anthelmintics, with no response and a mortality of virtually 100%. Usually, only a small number of lambs is affected.

Diagnosis

Without experience, the disease is easily missed unless there is post-mortem examination, where both kidneys are seen to be enlarged and very pale, and often haemorrhagic foci are seen in the abomasal mucosa. Histology shows a non-inflammatory nephrosis. Suspect cases should have a blood sample taken for urea concentration (often higher than 40 mmol/l, normal 6.5).

Treatment

Treatment with antibiotics, anthelmintics, anticoccidials and/or vitamin preparations have no effect.

Causes

Although there have been many suggestions as to possible causes, including a range of infections or toxic chemicals, the cause is unknown but the histology suggests a bacterial toxin, possibly from a clostridial organism.

Further reading
Angus, K K, Hodgson, J C, Hosie, B D, Low, J C, Mitchell, G B B, Dyson, D A and Hollman, A. 'Acute nephropathy in young lambs', *Veterinary Record*, Vol. 124, 9–14.

PNEUMONIA

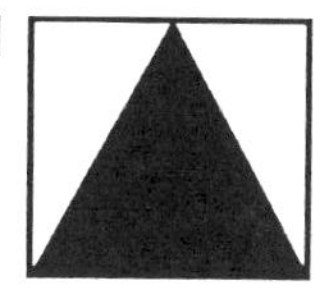

PASTEURELLOSIS

This is one of the most common causes of rapid/sudden death and of pneumonia in sheep. As most sheep carry the causal organism, *Pasteurella haemolytica*, in the naso-pharynx or tonsils, the mere isolation of this organism in nasal swabs or at PME, does not establish the diagnosis; it is generally held that it requires some stress factor or intercurrent disease to excite pasteurellosis.

There are three different manifestations of the disease:

(1) Septicaemia and rapid death in young lambs (few days to 3 months old).

(2) Pneumonia in older lambs and adults, most commonly in late spring and early summer (May–July) but also in store and fattening lambs in the autumn and winter.

(3) Septicaemia and rapid death in the fattening and store lamb (6–9 months old) in the autumn and winter (October–December).

Two biotypes of the organism can be distinguished: Biotype A is mainly involved in (1) and (2) and Biotype T in (3). There are at least 15 serotypes but 8 are responsible for the majority of clinical problems.

Clinical signs

(1) The most common first sign is one or two sheep found dead.

(2) A few others may appear very ill and separated from the rest and unwilling to be driven; they are usually febrile (over 40°C, 104°F) and have laboured respirations. Auscultation may be convincing but it can be difficult to be sure that pneumonia is the problem. Some may have crusted eyelids and nostrils and usually there is some coughing in the group. About 10% may become affected in an outbreak.

Diagnosis

(1) Try to find a predisposing reason for the deaths/illness; in particular, enquire if the group has been moved or handled in the last day or so, or whether the weather has been noticeably different, e.g. wet and windy (rain/windchill factor), or warm and still. Other intercurrent infections such as PI3 virus, Jaagsiekte and tick-borne fever may also predispose to clinical outbreaks.

(2) Consider clostridial diseases, in particular Pulpy Kidney and Braxy, and check on vaccination dates.

(3) Necropsy of fresh carcases. *P. haemolytica* needs to be isolated in large numbers to be sure and ask the VIC for sero-typing to check against the vaccine sero-types.

Treatment and control

Sometimes the group is large and inaccessible, which means the incidence is unsure, PME is delayed and there is a very real difficulty in deciding when to do something, i.e. gather (which may make matters worse) and treat (the lot?). Often an 'irritating' number of deaths occur over a period of days or weeks and then unaccountably cease.

(1) Rescue and isolate affected sheep. Treat these and as many contacts as seem worthwhile, with, for example, long-acting oxytetracycline, given twice at a 4 day interval.

(2) Look at the environmental conditions, e.g. wet, exposed, over-crowded, lush food, and consider providing plenty of shelter or moving the group, although the moving could make matters worse. In the long-term, avoid, if possible, very exposed wet and windy sites which induce stress and encourages the flock to crowd into small sheltered sites which, in turn, intensify the aerial spread of pathogens.

(3) Consider vaccination. Ovipast (Hoechst Animal Health), costing approx. 30p a dose, is a dead vaccine containing most of the sero-types known to cause disease, and requires two doses at approx. 4 weeks interval to provide useful protection. If given to ewes in late pregnancy it not only affords protection to the ewes that spring, when the incidence of enzootic pneumonia is highest, but also to the lambs via colostrum for the first few weeks of life and so helps to cover the first major risk period for pasteurella septicaemia. To cover adequately the next few weeks and months, lambs need to be given two doses of vaccine as soon as possible after birth; there is evidence that any colostrum-derived antibody does not interfere with the response to this early vaccination.

The position regarding vaccination has become somewhat compromised by the combining of this vaccine with a clostridial vaccine (Heptavac, Hoechst Animal Health), costing approximately 30p a dose to form the very popular product Heptavac-P (Hoechst Animal Health) costing approximately 40p per dose. Whilst such a combination is ideal for the vaccination of ewes, it matches the needs of lambs less well where clostridial protection via colostrum lasts for up to 16 weeks, whereas pasteurella protection lasts only 3–4 weeks. In practice, if this combination is to be used in flocks where there is a significant incidence of septicaemia and sudden deaths in young lambs which is diagnosed as pasteurellosis, the normal lamb clostridial vaccination schedule needs to be brought forward to 1 and 2 months rather than the usual 3 and 4 months.

Unfortunately, the vaccine does not appear to be as effective against the Biotype T and therefore appears to be less adequate in the control of pasteurellosis in the later store and fattening lamb.

PARASITIC PNEUMONIA (Husk)

Although sheep are commonly infected with a number of nematodes which are found in various parts of the respiratory system, the only species which is associated with clinical disease is *Dictyocaulus filaria*. It is found in the trachea and bronchi. The heaviest pasture infections with infective larvae occur from September to November. These larvae can overwinter and act as a source of infection to the next season's lambs.

The disease is not so important clinically as 'husk' in cattle which may be associated with the more frequent anthelmintic dosing of lambs for parasitic gastro-enteritis, which incidentally reduces the number of worms in the lungs. However, the worm is common and can cause coughing and loss in condition in lambs in August to October. The lambs develop a strong immunity and few worms are found in older sheep. Many lambs are sent to slaughter before the peak of infection.

Diagnosis

Diagnosis is based on clinical signs and seasonal incidence and can be confirmed by faecal examination for first stage larvae by the Baermann apparatus. Faeces should be fresh and *D.filaria* can be distinguished from the larvae of other non-pathogenic worms in that they are long (500um), have a blunt tail and a cephalic knob and contain refractile granules.

Treatment and control

All the modern benzimidazoles, levamisole and ivomectin are effective against *D.filaria* and can be used to treat clinically affected lambs. Parasitic bronchitis is unlikely to occur where these drugs are used earlier in the year to control parasitic gastro-enteritis but some drugs (e.g. oxibendazole, Widespec, Rycovet Ltd and thiophanate, Nemafax, RMB Animal Health Ltd) are effective against stomach and intestinal worms but not against *D.filaria* at the usual dose.

ATYPICAL PNEUMONIA

This is an unsatisfactory name given to the type of pneumonia which closely resembles that so commonly found in the fattening pig and housed calf. It is principally a disease problem in the housed or densely stocked fattening or store lamb (3 to 12 months old) and associated with a variety of agents such as *Mycoplasma ovipneumoniae*, parainfluenza virus type 3 (PI3) and adenovirus. It is particularly common following the mixing of lambs introduced from the market in autumn and winter.

Clinical signs

The disease is characterised by chronic coughing, ocular and nasal discharges, and is usually afebrile, although the occasional acute pneumonic lamb arises which is febrile, off food, listless, and with obvious respiratory distress; these cases are associated with *Pasteurella haemolytica* biotype A infection. Affected lambs take several weeks longer to reach slaughter weight and consume more food to do so.

Diagnosis

Based on the clinical signs, environmental conditions and the pathology of lungs at PME or slaughter.

Control

As for pigs and calves.

(1) Supply more fresh air.

(2) Reduce numbers under one roof, and in any one group.

(3) Split groups according to age, size and origin.

(4) Inject with long-acting oxytetracycline or tylosin.

(5) Consider pasteurella vaccination.

SLOW VIRAL PNEUMONIAS

Jaagsiekte or Sheep Pulmonary Adenomatosis (SPA) = Driving sickness

Although this condition has caused worrying losses in some flocks, particularly of Scottish origin where the incidence can be up to 10%, it usually only causes sporadic deaths, but its potential danger is illustrated by the losses that occurred in Iceland in housed sheep. It is a contagious adenomatous tumour of the lungs of sheep and possibly goats, and thought to be associated with a retro and/or herpes virus with an incubation period of up to 3 years.

Clinical signs

The signs are severe respiratory distress but without much coughing, in an individual adult sheep when driven. This respiratory embarrassment, which sounds like 'bubbly porridge', on auscultation, increases over several weeks and the sheep progressively loses weight. Characteristically, if the ewe is held with its head lowered, relatively large volumes (30–300ml) of clear mucous exudate flow from the nostrils; this fluid is infectious. There is no fever and the animal feeds up to the terminal stages when there is often fulminating pasteurellosis.

Diagnosis

There is no serological test and diagnosis is based on clinical signs and PME; the lungs may weigh up to 4kg (1.5kg is normal). It should be possible to test the tracheal fluid for the reverse transcriptase enzyme essential to the retrovirus. Jaagsiekte can predispose to pasteurellosis and so, where pasteurellosis appears a persistent problem in adult sheep, histology of the lungs is required.

Control

Prompt slaughter of the obviously affected. At present, the condition should be regarded as a potential problem rather than a real one, but housing sheep could alter the situation. Once a serological test becomes available, then monitoring and pre-clinical culling becomes a possibility. Jaagsiekte is included in the MAFF Sheep and Goat Health Scheme by means of abattoir monitoring (see page 105).

Maedi/Visna

For all practical purposes, this condition is similar to Jaagsiekte, although more recently introduced into the UK and only a few clinical cases have, as yet, been recorded. Maedi means 'air hunger' and it is seen as a chronic progressive pneumonia affecting sheep and goats over 3 years old and is invariably fatal. Visna,which means 'wasting', is the nervous form of the disease, and is seen as a progressive paralysis of the hind legs of adults. Both conditions are caused by the same lenti-virus, and is spread particularly indoors and via the colostrum, a risk that increases with the increasing popularity of colostrum 'banks'.

The disease, like Jaagsiekte, has, as yet, little significance to the commercial lamb producer, but with the increased housing of ewes the position may change. However, unlike Jaagsiekte, there are useful serological diagnostic tests which are used in the MAFF Sheep and Goat Health Scheme (see page 105). This has particular application for the pedigree breeder, not only for control within the flock, but for registered sales and for shows.

Clinical signs

Similar to Jaagsiekte but without the diagnostic flow of bronchial fluid.

Diagnosis

In the individual this is based on clinical signs and PME. Serological tests such as the agar gel precipitin test (AGPT) and enzyme-linked immunosorbent assay test (ELISA) at £2.50 a test are useful at the flock level, but false negative results, due to delay in production or immuno-suppression, do occur, which makes them less useful in the individual animal.

Control

(1) Slaughter the affected.

(2) Do not breed from the offspring of affected ewes.

(3) Keep a young flock and only keep replacements from the young ewes.

(4) Purchase from accredited flocks only.

(5) Join the Ministry scheme and eradicate by test and slaughter.

CEREAL PROBLEMS

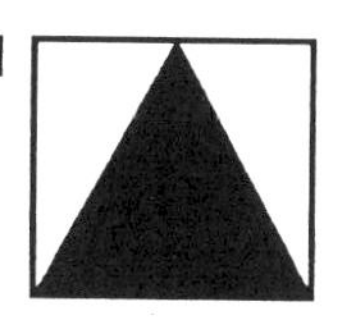

UROLITHIASIS

This is mainly a hazard for the housed 2 to 4 month old castrated male lamb fed a lot of concentrate.The fine sand-like calculi, usually consisting of magnesium phosphate, obstruct the penis either at the vermiform appendage or at the sigmoid flexure.

Clinical signs

(1) The lambs show discomfort with straining, kicking at the abdomen, twitching of the tail and general restlessness.

(2) A precipitate of crystals may be found on the preputial hairs which are often dry and sometimes bloodstained.

(3) 'Water belly' may occur, with urine leaking subcutaneously from a ruptured urethra, or into the abdominal cavity from a ruptured bladder.

Treatment *(not easy, but urgent)*

Depending on the severity and success –

(1) Spasmolytic and analgesic injection (e.g. Buscopan Compositum, Boehringer Ingelheim Ltd).

(2) Twice daily drenching (or tubing) with a litre of 0.9% ammonium or potassium chloride.

(3) Amputate the vermiform appendage with scissors; in young lambs it is still adherent.

(4) Perineal urethrotomy.

Control

(1) *When cases are occurring:*

(a) Change and reduce the amount of concentrate.

(b) Ensure plenty of fresh water.

(c) Supply salt (NaC1) as licks, or in ration or in drinking water.

(d) Add 2% ammonium chloride to the ration.

(e) Contact the food supplier.

(2) *In future:*

(a) Ensure no magnesium added to concentrates; do not exceed 200g Mg0/tonne.

(b) Ensure Calcium/Phosphorus ratio is approx. 2:1; include 1.5% ground limestone in the diet.

(c) Ensure minimum of 1% salt in concentrate.

(d) Ensure plenty of fresh water.

(e) Avoid castration.

RUMEN ACIDOSIS (Cereal overeating)

Following the fermentation of excessive starch, the rumen contents become acid and hypertonic leading to rumenitis, scouring, dehydration and acidosis. It frequently occurs when sheep are given too much cereal too quickly, particularly in the housed fattening or store lamb, but it occurs also in ewes when first housed and even when grazing barley stubble. Most frequently, there is just a short period of indigestion leading to scouring and dirty tails which self-cures. However, it can be much more serious with sheep 'found dead'.

Clinical signs

These appear about a day after excessive intake:

(1) Many of the group look a bit miserable, with dirty tails and soft to watery faeces, and reduced appetite.

(2) A few may be found dead or very ill, with diarrhoea, grinding teeth, sunken eyes, rapid respirations and recumbent.

Diagnosis

Is usually fairly obvious from seeing what has been fed and the clinical signs, but pulpy kidney and pasteurellosis should also be considered; atypical pneumonia may also be present in the group and this complicates the respiratory picture. PME shows an easily detached rumen epithelium with haemorrhagic sub-mucosa.The contents are sour-smelling and acid (below 5 is suspicious and below 4.5 is certain).

Treatment

Depending on how sick the lambs are:

(1) Drench with magnesium hydroxide mixture (10ml twice daily) or chalk (3g twice daily), and a bloat drench if tympanitic.

(2) One to two litres of glucose saline i/v, 10ml of 2.5% solution of sodium bicarbonate, and 5ml of B-complex vitamins (e.g. Parentrovite – Beecham Animal Health).

(3) Long-acting oxytetracycline i/m.

(4) Supply good quality hay and reduce the concentrates.

(5) Ensure plentiful fresh clean water.

Future control

(1) Introduce concentrates gradually over several days. Whole barley is less risky than if crushed or ground.

(2) Provide adequate good quality hay.

(3) Provide adequate trough space so that the greedy ones don't eat the lot.

(4) Ensure adequate water supply.

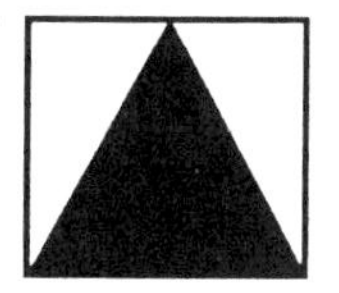

CONTAGIOUS OPHTHALMIA

Contagious Conjunctivokeratitis (CCK), Ovine Infectious Keratoconjunctivitis, (OIKC), Pink Eye, Heather Blindness.

This is a very common disturbance of sheep's eyes. Usually there is only superficial irritation recognisable by scleral congestion, lachrymation, blinking and some blepharospasm (grade 1). Some cases, however, particularly adult sheep, show corneal inflammation with blood vessels and pannus spreading from the corneo-scleral margin (grade (2), and progressing to shallow corneal ulceration and temporary blindness (grade 3). Both eyes are usually affected but not always simultaneously or to the same grade. Blind ewes get insufficient food and are accident-prone.

Outbreaks often arise after movement; this is probably because *Mycoplasma conjunctivae*, the organism most commonly associated with the disease, is spread by close sheep-to-sheep contact rather than by vector or airborne transmission. Bacteria such as *Branhamella ovis* and *Staphylococcus aureus* may play a role in increasing the ocular reaction, and *Chlamydia psittaci* has been isolated from some outbreaks.

Without treatment, the duration of the disease is very variable; if only the scleral is involved, complete resolution may occur in a day or so, but if the cornea is involved, inflammation may persist for 3 or 4 weeks. However, many carriers remain and relapses and new infections are frequent, with the result that the disease persists in the flock.

The disease causes discomfort and individual cases certainly merit treatment when there is obvious blepharospasm, which usually indicates corneal involvement. A single systemic injection of a long-acting oxytetracycline (e.g. Terramycin LA Injectable Solution, Pfizer Ltd) together with a tetracycline infusion into both eyes (e.g. Aureomycin Ophthalmic Ointment, Cyanamid UK) preferably twice daily for three days, are indicated. Separation from the group may be necessary in order to ensure proper care and treatment.

In an outbreak, it is worth considering injecting all the immediate contacts with oxytetracycline: this routine can also be applied to all newly purchased sheep, for example rams, in order to reduce the risk of importing fresh strains of *M.conjunctivae* into the flock.

The frequent movement and mixing of sheep are obvious hazards and should be kept to a minimum.

It is worth noting that this condition is very different in its aetiology, pathogenesis and severity, from so-called 'New Forest' disease in cattle, and that some ocular preparations, for example, the penicillins for use in cattle, are inappropriate for sheep.

BRIGHT BLINDNESS

(Clear blind, Glass-eyed)

This is an irreversible blindness in adult sheep,mainly reported in Yorks/Lancs flocks, but occurring in hill flocks in other areas. The condition affects both eyes equally and simultaneously. The retina shows progressive degeneration with atrophy of the rods and cones; the tapetal arteries and veins are narrowed and there is a marked green reflection from the tapetum. Ophthalmoscopic examination of the retina is easy because the pupils are dilated and the cornea and lens are clear.

The prevalence may be over 5% and usually becomes apparent in the autumn following the bracken season. It is caused by a toxic factor in bracken, and may require several seasons of bracken consumption before signs become apparent; it is therefore only seen in adult sheep.

As the condition is slowly progressive, the sheep have time to adapt and the blindness may only become apparent when the sheep are driven or placed in strange surroundings. They are not unwell, appearing perhaps more alert than usual and are not easy to catch. They are, however, more prone to accident and to get lost. They require culling.

ENTROPION

Entropion is common in new-born lambs, involving one or both lower eyelids. The incidence varies from flock to flock but cases occur in most flocks and many receive inadequate attention resulting in unnecessary discomfort and corneal damage. Some flocks have a distressing number of severe cases and there is sometimes good evidence to suggest a breed factor, with a recessive gene involvement.

Treatment

(1) Mild entropion can be easily everted by finger pressure, and is all that is required.

(2) More severe cases, where the lower-lid is turned-in a lot causing blepharospasm, keratitis and corneal ulceration, require more vigorous attention, such as:

(a) subcutaneous injection of a liquid below the margin of the lid, sufficient to produce a bleb which everts the lid. Liquid paraffin is effective, but an antibiotic preparation is more sensible (e.g. Streptopen injection, Coopers Pitman-Moore).

or

(b) Suture a tuck in the skin below the lid with 14 or 16mm Michel clips (Arnolds Veterinary Products).

Most cases merit antibiotic eye ointment at the time, and if possible for the next day or so.

Control

(1) Consider the breeding lines.

(2) Mark and record each case and don't breed from them.

SKIN AND WOOL DISORDERS

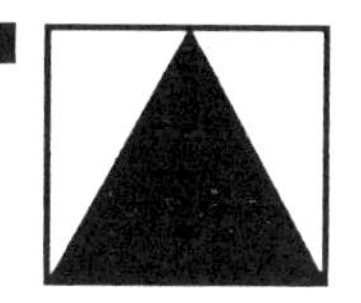

Although a number of specific conditions affect the skin and wool of sheep, it must be remembered that because the production of wool is an active process, many systemic diseases will result in local or generalised loss of wool.

DISORDERS ASSOCIATED WITH PRURITIS

The flock should be viewed from a distance to obtain some indication of the proportion of ewes showing signs of pruritis – restlessness, stamping of feet, rubbing against posts or nibbling or biting at areas of the body. Individual affected sheep should be examined to determine the areas affected, the nature of the lesion including involvement of the skin and specimens for further examination should be taken from active lesions.

(1) Parasitic conditions

Sheep scab, psoroptic mange (and other mites)

This notifiable disease is caused by a non-burrowing mite, a variety of *Psoroptes communis* which is specific for sheep. It is highly contagious, and is spread by direct contact, and is usually introduced by the purchase of sheep. The mites live on the skin surface and pierce the skin to feed on lymph. Rapidly extending moist lesions develop from the pustules at the site of feeding and the fleece becomes matted above these areas. Sheep show signs of extreme irritation and rub vigorously and nibble at the affected areas which are particularly over the shoulder and flanks. Extensive wool loss occurs, often extending, in neglected cases, to most of the body.

The mites are capable of enormous multiplication over a relatively short time with maximum numbers occurring 6–12 weeks after infection. The disease is most active during the winter but can be seen in summer, though latent infections with small numbers of mites are common in the summer, with a flare-up to typical disease in autumn and winter. Severe infections result in marked loss in condition and death.

In typical outbreaks of sheep scab, when a high proportion of the flock is affected and lesions are severe, diagnosis is straightforward since the white mites can just be seen with the naked eye. When mites are not so numerous, superficial skin scrapings should be taken from the edge of the lesion for microscopic examination.

A number of other mites are found on sheep, including *Chorioptes ovis*, usually on the legs, scrotum or brisket and Tyroglyphid or forage mites which can be found all over the body and which, though they are non-parasitic, occasionally cause pruritis. *Psoroptes* has well-developed legs which protrude beyond the body, and the legs of the first two pairs of legs, in both male and female mites, end in bell-shaped suckers which are on long segmented (the diagnostic feature) pedicels.

Any suspected outbreak must be reported to the Divisional Veterinary Officer, who will enforce compulsory dipping, institute movement restrictions and attempt to trace sheep onto and off the farm.

Sheep scab has been a notifiable disease in the UK for many years and was eradicated by compulsory dipping in 1952. Unfortunately, after years of freedom, new cases were diagnosed in 1973 and despite dipping regulations which have exerted some control, outbreaks have occurred every year.

The number of outbreaks has fallen from 157 in 1983 to 36 in 1988 but so far it has proved impossible to eradicate sheep scab. This is probably due to the much greater movement of sheep, the inefficient dipping of sheep and the lack of effective supervision by local authorities. Many cases have not been recognised by farmers since half the recent outbreaks were detected by government veterinary officers.

For the past 5 years the whole of the UK has been designated a control area and all sheep have had to be dipped in a scab-approved dip on two occasions - early summer and late autumn. The progress made was then reviewed and, for 1989, a single dipping period from September 24 to November 4 for the whole country was approved. It is likely that a similar recommendation will be made for 1990, but discussions are in progress between the MAFF and the sheep industry which may modify the scheme. The possibilities range from the present policy of compulsory dipping of all sheep, the designation of 'infected' and 'clean' areas or even the removal of sheep scab from the list of notifiable diseases, making its control a concern for each individual farm.

The scab-approved dips contain either organo-phosphorus compounds (e.g. diazinon, propetamphos) or a synthetic pyrethroid (flumethrin, Bayticol, Bayer UK Ltd). Concern has been expressed over the toxicity of OP compounds for those dipping the sheep. Sheep must be in the dip for 1 minute and must be completely submerged at least once. Concern has also been expressed that dipping in autumn during the tupping period would adversely affect reproductive performance but the limited amount of experimental studies do not support this contention.

Lice and keds

There are two types of lice, biting, *Damalinia ovis* and sucking, *Linognathus ovillus* and *L. pedalis*. The sheep ked, *Melophagus ovinus*, is a wingless fly and is now very rare in the UK. The life cycle of these highly host-specific insects is similar with all stages on the sheep. Adults live for only a few days off the sheep.

Clinical signs are similar with heavy infections leading to irritation involving a high proportion of the flock with resulting rubbing, nibbling and damage to fleece. Populations are highest in the winter months. Keds are large brown insects and are easily seen but lice may be difficult to see. A wadge of wool should be clipped from the edge of a lesion and examined in a bright light with a magnifying glass for adults and eggs attached to the wool.

Lice and keds are very susceptible to a range of insecticidal drugs including organo-phosporus compounds (e.g. diazinon) and synthetic pyrethroids (e.g. flumethrin, cypermethrin). Treatment is usually carried out in autumn or winter. The insecticides may be applied by dipping, spray races, jetting or 'pour-ons' and there is a residual activity in the fleece for several months. The injectable form of ivomectin is recommended for louse control in cattle but the oral preparation, licensed for sheep, is not.

Blowfly myiasis-fly strike

Strike is a common condition seen throughout the summer months in the UK in which larvae of *Lucilia sericata* (green bottle fly), *Phormia terrae-novae* (black blow fly) and *Calliphora erythrocephala* (blue bottle) invade the skin under soiled fleece resulting in extreme discomfort and rapidly leading to death. The most common areas which are affected are around the breech associated with soiling due to scouring, on the side of the body where fleece is contaminated from foot rot lesions when the sheep lie down and in various sites associated with wounds. Affected animals are restless, show vigorous wagging of the tail when the breech is affected or biting at affected areas and are often separated from the flock. The larvae of the flies, which develop within a few days from the eggs laid in the moist contaminated area, burrow into the skin and cause a foul-smelling wound. The lesions are typical but the maggots may not be easily seen as they will have burrowed into the wound. It is important that the flock should be examined at least once a day to detect early cases as affected animals die within a few days of the initial attack.

Affected areas should be clipped and the maggots removed physically. Diluted dip fluid is larvicidal and helps to protect the area against further strike. Since secondary bacterial infection is common, injections of antibiotic are valuable.

Control is by insecticidal treatment in the summer and one treatment is effective for two months. Most of the chemicals which have been described earlier for scab, lice and ked control are also effective against blowfly strike and a variety of formulations including pour-ons (e.g. cyromazine, Vetrazin, Ciba-Geigy) are available. Control of the factors predisposing to strike are also critically important.

Head-fly

This disease is caused by a non-biting muscid fly, *Hydrotaea irritans* which swarm around the head of sheep, causing it to rub its head which leads to self-trauma. The flies then feed on the exudate of blood and lymph, which leads to further attacks. The area where horns and skin join is often the site of small breaks in the skin which probably explains why the condition is virtually confined to horned breeds. The disease is most common in the North of England and South of Scotland but the fly occurs throughout the UK and we have seen the disease in North Wales in hornless sheep. The wounds do not heal whilst the flies are active and extensive lesions involving much of the skin of the head are produced. Loss in condition and disfigurement of the skin occurs.

The flies are active from late June until the end of September on still, warm humid days and there is only a single generation of flies each year. Non-feeding females rest in trees and can fly half a kilometre a day. Each female produces 1 or 2 batches of about 30 eggs which hatch to larvae in pasture soil (not dung) from September to May especially near woods. Pupae are found near the soil surface from May to June. The flies can feed on a variety of animals; meal analysis shows that about 80% feed on cattle.

Many methods of control have been tried but none is entirely successful. The most effective method appears to be the application to the top of the head and base of the horns of a synthetic pyrethroid insecticide (e.g. cypermethrin, Ovipor, Rycovet Ltd). In areas of high challenge, the treatment will have to be repeated monthly. Cypermethrin impregnated eartags tied *loosely* between the horns in order to allow movement provide considerable protection but not if used solely as an eartag. There is a 7-day withdrawal period for meat.

Ticks see page 77.

Further reading:
Appleyard, Bill and Bailie, Harry (1984). Parasitic skin diseases of sheep. *In Practice*, Vol. 6,4–9.
Tarry, D. (1986). The control of sheep headfly disease. *Proceedings of the Sheep Veterinary Society*. Vol. 11, 51–56.

<u>(2) Non-parasitic conditions</u>

Scrapie

Scrapie should be suspected when an individual adult sheep begins to rub, nibble or suck its fleece for no obvious reason, leading to bilateral semi-bald patches on its flanks, hind-legs, bridge of nose and top of head. The skin and fleece appear normal except for self-inflicted healing scabs. The irritation is increased by firm finger rubbing of the back and itchy areas. Other neurological signs are often present (and sometimes on their own) and there is a worsening over days/weeks. For further details see page 37.

DISORDERS WITH USUALLY LITTLE OR NO PRURITIS

<u>(1) Infectious</u>

Orf (Contagious Pustular Dermatitis [CPD], Scabby Mouth

This disease is a constant worry to sheep farmers as shown by the priority that they give it for further research. It threatens to develop into an outbreak and spread to the teats of ewes, which in turn can lead to both faulty suckling and mastitis. Occasional cases also inexplicably develop extensive and persistent lesions, and there is a risk of spread to the shepherds, particularly to those caring for orphan lambs, and the lesions on fingers, face or neck are, at best, irritating and painful, and at worst, there is a very marked reaction with local lymphatic involvement. The worry is compounded by the fact that present control measures are inadequate and the epidemiology of the condition remains unclear. However, whilst the appearance and siting of the lesions in and around the mouth suggest a lot of discomfort and interference with sucking and grazing, many lambs survive without problems, most cases self-cure in a few weeks and the incidence in most flocks remain low.

It is caused by a parapox virus which survives in dry scabs, from year to year indoors, but for shorter periods outside; small scabby lesions on the hairy areas of the face and limbs are also persistent sources of the virus; it is susceptible to iodophor disinfectants. It has a distinct shape and size and is easily recognised by electron microscopy (EM), although it is morphologically indistinguishable from the Paravaccinia (Pseudo-Cow pox) virus found in teat lesions of cattle. It has an affinity for hairy areas particularly at the weak junctions between skin and mucosae, eg. commissure of lips, but it requires some surface damage to allow invasion, e.g. splitting of lip.s, eruption of incisors, rough grazing, and teat sores following vigorous sucking and incisor injury by hungry lambs.

The lesions are characteristic and diagnostic, although when in doubt, unpreserved scabs should be sent to the VI Centre for EM examination. They start as raised red papules which coalesce and in a few days proceed through vesicles and pustules to thick scab formations which are firmly attached to what looks like exuberant granulation, and removal causes an awkward amount of haemmorhage. Secondary mixed bacterial infection is common and exaggerates the local response. The lesions are often confined to the outside of the lips and are sometimes barely noticeable, but in young lambs, granulomatous lesions are not uncommon within the mouth, involving the gums and sometimes the tongue. Despite their appearance, the lesions do not appear to cause much distress unless particularly exuberant and extensive, and whilst there may be some lambs who fail to thrive, most will self-cure within 3–6 weeks. The situation becomes much more serious, however, if and when the lesions secondarily arise on the teats of ewes.

Immunity following primary infection is incomplete and short-lived, perhaps only a few months, but subsequent infections are likely to produce milder lesions. It appears to rely on mediation by cells within the skin, and although circulating and lymphatic antibodies are produced, they are not protective, and therefore neither is colostrum.

A live vaccine is available (Scabivax, Coopers Pitman-Moore) costing about 25p a dose. It is applied by skin scarification, usually on the hairless area of the inner thigh. Its efficacy and timing is debatable but it probably shortens recovery time if not preventing infection. It is commonly applied to ewes in early or mid pregnancy, especially to those which will be housed at lambing, in an attempt to reduce the weight of infection in carriers, and to protect the teats. It is sometimes applied to lambs in the summer a few weeks before sale, in an attempt to avoid lip lesions and subsequent refusal at markets. It is also sometimes applied to young lambs in contact with infections, or where there has been a previous history of disease, and even to those with lesions, in an attempt to prevent or control an outbreak; the consensus seems to be that this should be a last rather than a first resort. It certainly should be not be used on ewes within six weeks of lambing nor in flocks that have no history of the disease, as the induced scabs are a source of further infection. The vaccine, like the natural infection, needs to be handled with care.

Individual severe cases should be separated to ensure proper nursing and daily application of antibiotic. Ewes should be inspected for teat lesions, and it may be necessary to wean and hand-rear their lambs (but be careful!), and to dry-off the ewe following infusion of long-acting antibiotic. Where necessary, sheep should also be removed from pastures that appear to be causing face or limb abrasions, e.g. thistles. Where possible, contaminated pens should be cleaned out and disinfected with FAM before re-use, and again at the end of housing.

Strawberry Foot Rot

Occasionally lambs at pasture, often in wet, muddy and abrasive conditions, develop orf-like granulomas on the skin of the lower limbs particularly around the coronary bands, making the lambs obviously lame. The condition does not involve the foot and has no resemblance to foot rot, but the granulation tissue is likened to a strawberry! Orf virus particles can usually be isolated from the scabs, but so also can *Dermatophilus congolensis*, the organism more commonly associated with Lumpy Wool; it is uncertain which gets there first! Treatment should be for both, which means local dressing and systemic penicillin and streptomycin. The lambs need to be removed to dry pasture or housed. Some cases are particularly persistent and extensive, like other forms of orf, and these require euthanasia.

Ulcerative Balanoposthitis (Pizzle Rot) and Ulcerative Vulvitis

It is quite common to find a scabby ulcerative lesion at the junction of the skin and mucosa of the prepuce in rams and vulva in ewes. Raw, bleeding tissue is exposed if the scabs are removed, rather like orf, but the lesion is ulcerative rather than proliferative and it is unusual to find orf virus particles. In some cases in rams, the ulceration is confined to the glans penis and therefore goes unnoticed. The incidence can be quite high and is sometimes associated with tupping-time, suggesting venereal transmission.

Most cases self-cure or remain as minor lesions and there is no interference with breeding or fertility. However, occasionally the lesion are extensive with swelling, superficial sepsis and necrosis; in rams this may mean the involvement of both the glans penis and the mucosa of the sheath which becomes noticeably pendulous; subsequent scar tissue may interfere with future breeding.

The cause is still uncertain. Antibiotic aerosol spray is adequate for mild cases, but the more severe ones require systemic antibiotic and frequent local dressing and irrigation.

Staphylococcal folliculitis

Small discrete pustules are often seen around the lips, muzzles and under the tails of very young lambs, and on the udder of ewes (mammary impetigo). The surrounding skin is hyperaemic but not proliferative as is orf, and a crater is left when the pustules rupture, which heal quickly leaving a white patch if the skin is pigmented. Treatment is rarely necessary although local dressing and antibiotics directed at the causal organism, haemolytic coagulase positive *Staphylococcus aureus*, may occasionally be justified. It is worth remembering that this organism is a common cause of post-partum gangrenous mastitis, although the two conditions have not yet been linked.

Staphylococcal dermatitis (Facial or Periorbital dermatitis or eczema)

This is another variant of the skin lesions associated with *Staphylococcus aureus*. Extensive, suppurating scabby lesions are seen over the bony prominence of the orbit and face of sheep feeding at confined sites, typically late-pregnant ewes being fed concentrates with insufficient trough space, where they both injure themselves and each other, and transmit the infection to one another. Removal from the source of the problems and treatment with local dressing and antibiotics usually leads to rapid improvement, although serious and disfiguring complications can arise from eye involvement and from scar tissue. In future, adequate trough space must be provided (at least 45cm or 18in per ewe) and the food spread evenly and quickly to minimise aggression.

Mycotic dermatitis (Lumpy Wool)

This condition occurs in many if not most flocks, but generally as a low-grade self-limiting infection, and of little consequence other than some down-grading of the fleece. However, occasional outbreaks occur where the infection becomes more active and extensive, and secondary problem arise such as fly-strike; treatment is then necessary and in some flocks the condition requires routine control measures.

It is an exudative dermatitis passing rapidly through the stages of hyperaemia, exudate and scab. It is caused by an actinomycete *Dermatophilus congolensis* which also infects other species, e.g. horses, cattle and occasionally humans, and can remain viable in dry scabs for many months. It induces only weak local immunity, all of which means that successive 'attacks' are common and eradication is not an option.

The condition is often only noticed when a sheep is handled e.g. condition scored, and on parting the fleece, bundles of wool fibres are seen matted together by rough scabs. These scabs originate from the skin and are carried up in the growing fleece, eventually working to the tips and breaking off. The back and top sides of sheep are most commonly affected as these are the sites which get soaked following heavy rain or dipping; fat, flat-backed, close-woolled sheep are the most susceptible, where the fleece acts as a sponge. Other areas do get infected, appearing as scabs on the ears, head and limbs and scrotum of rams, and these are constant sources of re-infection elsewhere.

The distribution of the scabs and the general lack of pruritis are usually sufficiently diagnostic but if there is doubt, impression smears should be made of skin exudate or scabs taken, preferably those close to an active lesion, for laboratory examination.

Significant outbreaks usually follow wet weather or dipping, but it can also follow shearing when skin wounds may admit infection, and the skin surface is exposed to sunlight and general insult.

Sheep that need treatment should be housed and given either a 5 day course of a conventional dose or a single high dose (70mg/kg) of penicillin and streptomycin, e.g. 15ml of Streptopen Injection (Coopers Pitman-Moore); topical dressing with alum powder (MD Dusting Powder, Coopers Pitman-Moore) is also justified to prevent further surface spread. Where there is a continual problem in a flock, combined insecticidal and antimycotic dips are indicated (eg. MD Powder Dip, Coopers Pitman-Moore and Youngs Mycotic Dip, Youngs Animal Health Ltd.), especially immediately after shearing.

Fleece Rot (Canary Stain)

This is a variant of Mycotic Dermatitis and has a similar epidemiology, treatment and control. In this condition, the scabs are particularly colourful, commonly yellow but sometimes greenish-blue or brown, and follow infection by pigment-producing bacteria such as *Pseudomonas aeruginosa,* which may be primary skin invaders or secondary to dermatophilus.

Ringworm

This is an unusual condition in sheep, perhaps because of lack of contact with other hosts such as cattle or because of the protective fleece but housed shorn-ewes occasionally develop the condition, particularly if housed in buildings also occupied by cattle. It is caused by the fungus *Trichophyton verrucosum,* and on the hairy areas of head and face, it looks just like the condition in cattle, but the infection in the woolly areas often produces more obvious circular raised plaques which eventually lift off leaving the more typical crusty skin beneath.

Griseofulven is not licensed for use in sheep, and in any case, like cattle, it cannot be fed to pregnant stock, the group of sheep that appear to be the most vulnerable. The condition usually has to run its course, waiting for immunity and turn-out; topical iodine sprays may be useful but handle with care!

(2) Non-infectious

Wool Break and Wool Slip

A wool break usually follows any severe or prolonged debilitating condition including inadequate nutrition and is most marked during pregnancy and lactation. It is common to see ewes, often in poor condition, in late winter or spring patchily shedding their complete fleece and in the process looking very 'moth eaten'. Underneath, the skin is normal and providing the precipitating factors are reversed, normal wool regrows.

An allied but specific condition now known as Wool Slip, is frequently seen in housed, shorn ewes. Here, there is patchy loss of wool mainly confined to the hind quarters and back, developing within a few weeks of shearing. It is thought to be related to the stress of housing, shearing and cold, resulting in raised blood cortisol concentrations. The ewes are not obviously affected but it can lead to delay in turn-out.

Sunburn

Occasional cases of sunburn follow exposure to bright sunlight particularly recently shorn white-faced breeds. Marked skin erythema and oedema develop in exposed surfaces such as the back and udder, and necrosis with extensive scabs may develop. Affected sheep need housing and if secondary infection is suspected, e.g. dermatophilus, antibiotic therapy is indicated. Shade will be required in future.

Photosentisation (Yellowses)

Bright sunlight can also induce photosentisation if the white sheep have been previously eating a photodynamic agent as found, for example, in St John's Wort, or they have raised circulating concentrations of the photodynamic agent phylloerythrin, which arises when liver function is impaired. This impaired liver function can be caused by a variety of factors including toxic plants and fungi, and some drugs, so the precise factor is rarely discovered, particularly if only one or two sheep in a flock are involved.

The most noticeable feature is the marked oedema of the head and face including the eyelids and ears, which makes the sheep look very 'droopy' and miserable; other pigmented areas may also be affected and if severe enough, there is necrosis and eventual sloughing, particularly of the tips of the ears which then look 'cropped'.

Cases should be housed and carefully nursed. Blood samples for liver enzyme estimations may help to disclose the prognosis. If cases continue in a flock, a serious look for toxic plants is indicated and close questioning about recent treatments. There is some evidence that certain families are particularly susceptible.

Further reading:
G. B. B. Mitchell (1988). 'Non-parasitic skin diseases of sheep'. *In Practice,* Vol. 10, 69–73.
Self Assessment (1977). *In Practice,* Vol. 9, 92–93.

National health schemes
Individual farm health schemes
Sheep farm visit – check list
Farm questionnaire
An example of a health programme
Systematic examination of a sick ewe

SHEEP HEALTH SCHEMES

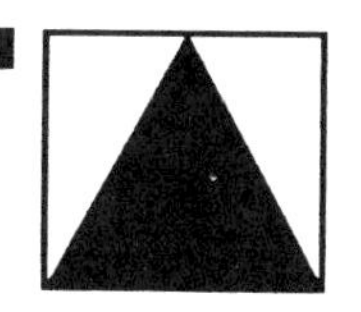

There are two major types of sheep health schemes- national and individual farm. The national schemes, which involve government veterinary officials, aim to produce a pool of sheep flocks of recognised health status with regard to certain specified diseases. Individual farm schemes are provided by practising veterinary surgeons for their clients and are 'tailor-made' for a particular flock.

NATIONAL HEALTH SCHEMES

There are two official schemes in the UK, each with a specific purpose:

(1) The Sheep and Goat Health Scheme, run by MAFF, is available throughout Britain. It started as an accreditation scheme for the control of maedi/visna (MV) and has been extended to include monitoring for enzootic abortion (EAE), scrapie and jaagsiekte. There are two categories of membership: Category I - MV accreditation and optional monitoring for the other diseases; Category II – monitoring for EAE only. This category is not available in Scotland where there is a similar scheme (see 2.). MV accreditation is based on a system of serological testing on all or a proportion of the flock, depending on whether it is 'open' or 'closed', and on the observation of rules concerning isolation, movement control and records. In 1989, 3511 flocks were accredited for MV in Category I of the scheme with 245 more undergoing qualifying tests. Monitoring for EAE is based on serology after lambing and the notification and testing of all abortions, and for scrapie and jaagsiekte on clinical examination and inspection of culled ewes at the slaughterhouse. 254 flocks have opted for EAE testing in Category I and 87 more are in Category II only.

Although there are obvious limitations to this scheme, it provides some evidence of health status to breeders, which may be sought (at a financial premium) by purchasers at home and, particularly, from abroad.

Costs vary with flock size, but for a 500 ewe open flock, MV testing would cost £1800 in the first year (2 tests of all ewes), £900 in the second year (1 test) and £250 in later years (1 test for 130 ewes). These fees do not include the cost of blood sampling but include all laboratory tests. EAE monitoring would cost annually about £1000 and scrapie and jaagsiekte about £200 each. A detailed schedule of the scheme is available from MAFF Offices.

(2) The Premium Health Scheme for Sheep Flocks, run by the Scottish Agricultural Colleges, is obviously only available in Scotland! The purpose of the scheme is to establish a register of commercial flocks with a high health status based on freedom from EAE and possessing vaccinal immunity to clostridial diseases and pasteurellosis. It is of particular value in providing halfbred replacements for lowland farms from hill flocks which are members of the scheme. EAE monitoring is by examination of all abortions, and by serology on all aborting and barren ewes and a sample of the healthy ewes. Flocks are categorised as closed, open low-risk and open high-risk, depending on the source of replacement stock. After 2 years of negative tests, a flock is 'certified' and included on a register. Every consignment of breeding stock from a certified flock is given a certificate indicating 'Premium Health Status' and a premium can be expected from purchasers for this status. The scheme has been particularly successful in the North of Scotland due to a farmer-led group encouraging participation. Over 250 000 ewes are involved in Caithness.

All lambs for sale must have received a course of vaccination injections for clostridial diseases and for pasteurellosis.

The annual costs of EAE monitoring for an open high-risk flock of 500 ewes would be about £625 excluding the fee for blood sampling.

Details may be obtained from the Scottish Veterinary Investigation Service.

INDIVIDUAL FARM HEALTH SCHEMES

Many sheep farmers are requesting advice from their veterinary surgeons on the formulation of health programmes. We reproduce here our approach to this opportunity, which is similar to those produced by others (e.g. Hindson, J. (1982), 'Sheep health schemes', *In Practice*, Vol. 4, 53–58; and Hindson, J (1989), 'Examination of the sheep flock before tupping', *In Practice*, Vol. 2, 149–55).

OBJECTIVE

To produce, monitor and maintain a unique health scheme for a particular farm, in the belief that this will both decrease disease and increase production.

THE SCHEME

The scheme has three components:

(1) A written Health Programme containing recommendations for the control of expected diseases and to improve production.

(2) Planned visits (3–6 annually) to monitor health and production.

(3) Reactions to events and to advise on new advances during the year, to keep the programme up-to-date.

Its success hinges on the degree of cooperation between the farmer and the practising veterinary surgeon and other advisers, and requires honest pooling of information.

(1) Health Programme

This programme is in the form of a diary and is tailor-made to suit the needs of the farm, following full discussion at the first visit. It is based around the farmer's proposed dates for tupping, housing, lambing and weaning, and includes dates for some or all of the following, depending on needs:

(a) Tupping – including early breeding, synchronisation, AI and ram testing.

(b) Condition scoring of ewes.

(c) Vaccination against clostridia, orf, abortion, foot rot, pasteurellosis.

(d) Dosing for copper, cobalt and selenium/Vit. E deficiencies.

(e) Worming for roundworms.

(f) Fluke drenching.

(g) Treatment for coccidiosis.

(h) Tapeworm treatment of dogs.

(i) Feeding and food analysis.

(2) Planned Visits

Several visits will be needed in order to assess the application and usefulness of the Health Programme. In the first year, six visits will usually be necessary according to the following plan; in subsequent years, fewer visits and samples are likely to be required.

Plan of visits to produce and monitor health programme

Date of visit (approx)		Jobs (some or all)	Time (approx) (for 500–1000 ewe flock)
VISIT 1*	Two months before tupping	1 Rams (all): Condition score, check fertility and feet. Ensure that the farmer/shepherd is able to condition score rams and ewes 2 Ewes (100 selected) Condition score, cull (teeth, age, udders) 3 Store lambs (a selection): Condition score 4 Take samples of blood and faeces for copper, B12, selenium, fluke and worms and abortion profile (Toxoplasma and Enzootic) 5 Check hay or silage and take samples for fibre, protein and energy estimates 6 Inspect pasture, examine for snail habitats 7 Check and discuss Farm Questionnaire (sent and hopefully returned in advance) 8 Discuss 'clean grazing' 9 Discuss farmer's objectives and possible targets for production	3 hours

Prepare draft programme following this visit and receipt of laboratory results

VISIT 2	Approx 1 month later	Discuss draft programme with farmer and finalise programme	1 hour
VISIT 3*	6 weeks before lambing	Condition score 100 ewes Advise about feeding (including trace elements) Treat clinical cases	1 hour
VISIT 4	2 weeks before lambing	Condition score 100 ewes Advise about housing facilities, colostrum, lambing and recording Treat clinical cases	1 hour
VISIT 5*	At peak lambing time	Clinical events Recording of lambs Advise about hypothermia and starvation, *E.coli*, coccidia and worming	1 hour
VISIT 6	12 weeks after lambing	Check growth rates	1 hour
		Total	8 hours

Notes
When more than one flock is involved with widely different lambing dates, more than 6 visits will be necessary, although it is probable that some can be combined. In addition to the 6 planned visits, advice will be available by phone.

* Visits in subsequent years

Possible charges

First Year (October 1989 prices)

1 For 6 visits	8 hours @ £30 per hour	£240.00
2 Laboratory services e.g.	12 bloods for mineral trace element profile	£70.00
	12 faeces for fluke	£36.00
	12 faeces for roundworm eggs	£42.00
	12 separate necropsies	£120.00
	2 food analyses	£40.00

These tests need not be applied routinely and may be reduced due to information obtained from clinical records from the farm.

(3) Reactions to events

It may be necessary to modify the original Health programme from time to time during the year, following informationobtained during and in between the planned visits. Information obtained about some or all of the following will be carefully considered:

(1) Breeds, ages and flock numbers.

(2) Condition of sheep.

(3) Quality and quantity of food.

(4) Housing arrangements.

(5) Lambing arrangements.

(6) Survey of snail habitats and drainage schemes.

(7) Pasture and grazing management.

(8) Clinical disease, e.g. pregnancy toxaemia, abortions, lameness, lamb losses, pneumonia.

(9) Laboratory findings, including post-mortem examination of a sufficient number of carcases to establish the cause of disease.

The programme will need amendment at the end of each year to incorporate new research, drugs, vaccines in the light of the experience of the past year and any alteration in the aims of the farmer.

Sheep farm visit Check list – farm/farmer

It is useful to have a checklist, particularly for the first visit, along the following lines

	Observations
(1) Geography	
(2) Geology	
(3) Climate	
(4) Possibilities for	Ticks
	Fluke
(5) Economic position	Income from sheep
	Income from other sources
	Gross margin/ewe
	Gross margin/ha
(6) Drugs and instruments (have a good look around)	
(7) Disease control measures (what's wrong with them?)	
(8) Welfare/care of sick	
(9) Labour/dogs (particularly availability of labour at lambing time)	
(10) Use of	Vets
	ADAS
	Commercial reps
	ATB

Sheep farm visit Check list – the sheep

	Observations
(1) General look at each flock/age group	Number of flocks
	Variety of breeds
	Extensive/intensive
	General condition
	Lameness
	Coughing
	Dirty tails
	Wool break
(2) Examine (handle) (a) 10% (or minimum of 50) ewes of each flock/age group	Condition score
	Teeth/age
	Blood sample (if necessary)
	(i) Abortion 'profile', ie. EAE/Toxoplasma
	(ii) Deficiencies
	Faecal sample (if necessary and from appropriate animals)
	(i) Fluke
	(ii) Worms
	(iii) Coccidia
(b) Clinical cases	Very thin
	Very lame
	Very sick
	Very nervous/depressed
	Very 'moth-eaten'
	Very dirty-tailed
	Tail end lambs
(c) Rams (all)	Condition score
	Feet
	Genitalia
	Faeces
(3) Abortions	Samples
(4) Suitable carcases	For PME

Sheep farm visit Check list – the food

	Observations
(1) Stocking rate (ewes/ha)	
(2) Quantity and quality of grazing	
(3) Reclamation/fertilisation	
(4) History of deficiency diseases	
(5) Mineral supplementation (food and dosing)	
(6) Stored roughage (hay, silage)	quantity/quality
(7) Concentrates	menu and quantity per ewe/day
(8) Storage of concentrates (and cats!)	
(9) Rack and trough space/ewe	
(10) Colostrum (source and quantity)	

Sheep farm visit Check list – the shelter

	Observations
(1) State of repair	
(2) Size/space/stocking density (ewes/sq m)	
(3) Atmosphere	
(4) Bedding	
(5) Water supply	
(6) Lighting	
(7) Trough space/ewe	
(8) Lambing pens	Numbers
	Cleanliness
	Heating
	Risks
	Lambing and revival kit
	Drugs
(9) The sheep	Puffing/blowing/coughing
	'Sweating' (if not shorn)
	Cleanliness
	Lameness
(10) Isolation facilities e.g. abortions/sick	

Farm questionnaire

(Sent in advance of visit 1 with a request to be returned 7 days before the visit. The questionnaire will be completed in June–August, depending on tupping dates)

Date	Farmer's name
	Address
	Telephone
Veterinary surgeon (for sheep consultant only)	Address
	Telephone
General information	total area (ha)
	total grassland
	silage
	hay
	roots
	home produced oats/barley for sheep
	other stock beside sheep
	labour available
	tenant/owner
	is there a large scale map of farm available?

Flock information

Total number of ewes

Total number of flocks

(A flock is a group of sheep with an identity! i.e. lambing date, pedigree, special purpose. If a group of sheep has a planned lambing date a month or more apart, treat as a separate flock.) Since a sheep year normally commences at tupping (Summer/Autumn) and concludes with lamb sales about 12 months later, the information requested should refer to the ewes and their lamb crop.

	Flock 1	Flock 2	Flock 3
Breed of ewe			
Number of ewes excluding ewe lambs			
Ewe lambs			
number			
age at tupping			
Breed of rams			
Number of rams			
Tupping date			
Lambing date			
Shearing date			
Dipping date			
Weaning date			
Housing date			
Wintered away dates			
Ewe feeding			
what			
when			
how much			
Dock/castrate			
how			
when			
Where lambed			
Is clean grazing available at turn-out i.e. not grazed by sheep the year before			
Is clean grazing available in July i.e. not grazed by sheep this year			
Lamb sales			
where			
when			
Purpose of flock			
Special practices (e.g. synchronisation, AI, scanning)			
Ewes purchased			
age			
source			
Percentage of flock lambed over 4 week period			

Disease control

	With what	To what	When
Vaccination			
Clostridia			
Pasteurella			
Foot rot			
Orf			
Any others			
Minerals			
Copper			
Cobalt			
Selenium			
Parasites			
Worms			
Fluke			
Coccidia			
Others			
Footbathing			
Condition scoring			
Tape-worm dosing to dogs			
Clinical problems encountered			
Ewes			
Lambs			
Laboratory reports			
What do you think is your most important problem?			

Production figures

Lambs	Flock 1	Flock 2	Flock 3
Number of lambs			
Born alive			
Born dead			
Dying in first 7 days			
Sold for slaughter before weaning			
Weaned			
Sold for slaughter after weaning			
Sold as stores			
Retained as stores			
Retained for breeding			

Lambs sold for slaughter

Month	Number	Average edcw in kg	Average price (state whether including variable premium)

Ewes	Number	When	Why
Died			
Culled			
Sold			
Purchased			

An example of a health programme

MONTH	VISIT	FLOCK 1: 85 ewes	FLOCK 2: 33 ewe lambs
SEPTEMBER	VISIT 1	**check ewes and rams** condition score feed feet footbath Footvax culling **ewes** blocks with monensin	
OCTOBER		10th TUP	**check ewes and rams** condition score feed feet footbath Footvax culling **ewes** blocks with monensin
NOVEMBER		**ewes** Footvax footbath	5th TUP
DECEMBER	VISIT 2	**ewes** house shear footbath worm condition score	**ewes** Footvax footbath
JANUARY	VISIT 3	**ewes and rams** Heptavac P condition score lambing kit pens	**ewes** house shear footbath worm condition score
FEBRUARY	VISIT 4	**LAMBING** **lambs** decoquinate in creep feed from 2 weeks	
MARCH			**ewes** Heptavac P condition score lambing kit pens
APRIL	VISIT 5	**TURN OUT** **ewes** Footvax	**LAMBING TURN OUT** **lambs** decoquinate in creep feed from 2 weeks **ewes** Footvax
		3 WEEKS **ewes** worm	3 WEEKS **ewes** worm
MAY	VISIT 6	3 WEEKS **ewes and lambs** worm	3 WEEKS **ewes and lambs** worm
JUNE		3 WEEKS **lambs** worm Heptavac P Footvax	
JULY		**WEAN**	**lambs** Heptavac P Footvax
AUGUST		**lambs** Heptavac P	**WEAN** **lambs** Heptavac P Footvax

Systematic examination of a sick ewe
A checklist for faults

(In order and stop when necessary to examine in more detail)

(1)	FROM A DISTANCE BEFORE HANDLING	
	Grade of Illness	(1) Mild, severe, dying
		(2) Acute, chronic
	General appearance	Excitable, depressed
	Fleece	Broken, 'bald' patches, rubbing, dirty tail
	Condition	Fat, thin
	Faeces	Loose, absent
	Respiratory	Distressed, very fast, very deep, coughing, nasal discharge
	Head	Held high/low, tilt/aversion, tremor, facial paralysis, dribbling
	Eyes (one or both)	Blinking, blepharospasm, discharges, cornea clear or cloudy
	Feeding	Poor appetite, off food, hungry, with difficulty
	Mobility	Unwilling to move, ataxic, recumbent, circles, lame (one or more limbs)
(2)	ON HANDLING	Difficult or easy to catch
	<u>(a) Standing</u>	Restrained with hind end in corner, facing light, standing astride
	Condition Score	1–5
	Fleece/skin	Wool break, ectoparasites, itchy (rub test), lumpy, scabs, sores, scars
	Age/teeth	Incisors – numbers of temporary/permanent, broken, over/under shot Molars – Feel face and ramus for lumps, pain. Look (gag) for gaps, loose, irregularities, food impaction
	Eyes (one or both)	Blind (Menace test), sclera pale or congested, grade of keratitis
	Cranial Nerves:	V& VII – Movement and sensation (eyelids, face, lips, gums)
	Temperature	Above 40°C (104°F)
	Pulse (femoral)	Strong/weak, very rapid, recovery
	Faeces	Dry pellets, soft, scour, smell
	Vulva/vagina	Discharge, membranes, smell , injury
	Joints/limbs (carpus, hock, stifle, hip)	Pain, swelling, stiff, abrasions, wasting
	Auscultation	Heart – rate and sounds, lungs – bubble and squeaks, rumen movements
	<u>(b) Tipped up</u>	Sitting comfortably on its tail,with back between legs of examiner
	Uterus	Abdominal distension, ballot, auscultate
	Udder	Swelling (2A, 2C or 3), milk/colostrum, teat sores/injury or blind
	Feet	Interdigital growths/sores, overgrowth, under-running, smell, pain (one or both claws), coronary band swelling/sinus
	Urine (by smothering or catheter)	Colour, turbidity, clinitest stick

Professional development

SHEEP VETERINARY SOCIETY

This is a specialist division of the British Veterinary Association and membership is open to all members of the veterinary profession (whether BVA members or not) and others interested in sheep. The Society holds two meetings a year (normally 2 or 3 days) in April and September which include farm visits as well as lectures and discussions in a friendly atmosphere. Membership is a 'must' for all who wish to keep up with developments in sheep veterinary work.
The Secretary
Dr Mike Sharp
Moredun Institute
Gilmerton Road
Edinburgh
EH17 7JH
is always pleased to hear from potential members. The annual membership fee is £5.00.

SPECIALIST QUALIFICATIONS OF THE ROYAL COLLEGE OF VETERINARY SURGEONS

In 1985, the Specialisation and Further Education Committee of the RCVS recommended that a Certificate and Diploma in Sheep Health and Production should be established as part of the programme to encourage members of the veterinary profession to study further in order to provide a better service for sheep farmers.
The syllabus covers the whole range of sheep husbandry and medicine, including Structure and Economics of the Sheep Industry, Reproduction and Breeding, Nutrition, Diseases and Health Programmes. The Certificate is designed for those in general veterinary practice who have more than an average interest in sheep and are willing to study a little more widely. The Diploma, also designed for those in practice who are willing to study a lot more (!), is stated as being 'of a high standard which will prove a tough hurdle totally different in concept from the relatively straightforward Certificate examination'. Details of syllabuses, regulations and fees are available from
RCVS
32 Belgrave Square
London
SW2X 8QP

Further reading

Hindson, J C and Winter, A C (1990). *An outline of clinical diagnosis in sheep.* Blackwell Scientific Publications.
Martin, W B. *Diseases of sheep.* Blackwell Scientific Publications (2nd edition due shortly).

INDEX